Unlearning
Migraine

Arturo & Inés
Goicoechea

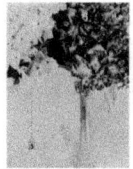

UNLEARNING MIGRAINE

© Arturo & Inés Goicoechea (2019)
Cover design: © V. Tellería, on a drawing by Inés Goicoechea ©1994
Edition: V. Tellería - I. Goicoechea (August 2019)
Illustrations and references: I. Goicoechea (2019)

ISBN: 9781082399206

Table of contents

Introduction

EXPERTS SAY THAT migraine is a genetic brain disease, of unclear origin, and irreversible. According to them, there would be neuronal centers, the "migraine generators", with a degree of pathological excitability, which would be activated spontaneously or by triggers. They state that the only way to alleviate the burden of suffering and disability (imposed by the inherited condition, they say) would be to lead an orderly life, identify and avoid the triggers and place oneself in the hands of a neurologist, who would prescribe painkillers to stop each crisis early and, optionally, a preventive treatment aimed at controlling the "hyperexcitability condition".

In *Unlearning Migraine*, I expose a contrasting and novel hypothesis: migraine is not transmitted by genes but is the consequence of the Neuroimmune System's learning process, a process tutored by expert information, with alarmist and sensitizing content. It would be part of an extensive section of

Pathology for which I propose the denomination of "autoneuro-immune diseases", characterized by the activation of unjustified states of alertness-protection.

From this perspective, the learned can also be unlearned, through the understanding of the biological plot of the migraine state and the re-exposure to normal activity.

ARTURO GOICOECHEA URIARTE

NEUROLOGIST. BORN IN Mondragón, Guipúzcoa, Spain, in 1946. Head of the Neurology Service at the Hospital Santiago in Vitoria, Spain, until 2011, currently retired. He remains active as a teacher and disseminator of the application of Neuroscience to the field of Neurology. He focuses on migraine and chronic pain, giving courses and talks and, for a decade or so, through his blog. All of this can be accessed at: arturogoicoechea.com.

Books published: *Jaqueca* ("Headache"), 2004. *Depresión y dolor* ("Depression and pain"), 2006. *Cerebro y dolor* ("Brain and pain"), 2008. *Migraña, una pesadilla cerebral* ("Migraine, a brain nightmare"), 2009.

INÉS GOICOECHEA TELLERÍA

Doctor in electronic engineering. Interested in the intersection of technology and neuroscience, in its dissemination, and empirical researcher of her own brain.

1 A PERFECT STUDENT

Montse is a good student. I met her at one of our courses for migraine patients. She had learned the lesson well and, together with her daughters, did a good job of unlearning everything she had learned. She "migrained" and "demigrained" precisely because of that: because she was a good student.
I asked her to contribute her experience to kickstart this book.

WHEN DR. GOICOECHEA asked me to write the preface to this book I was flattered. I owe him a lot, because thanks to his teachings I no longer suffer from migraines.

However, I was filled with a feeling of restlessness, the fruit of the responsibility that came with writing something that could rise to the occasion. What could I write? "Just tell your story," he said.

My story is neither original nor exciting. It is probably similar to that of many of you who are reading this and suffer or have suffered from migraine. It is one more story, full of ups and downs, of hard and unpleasant moments, of pilgrimage for medical consultations, of hope and hopelessness... but, above all, it is a story with a happy ending. I hope from the bottom of my heart that it can serve as an inspiration to someone to get rid of the nightmare of migraines.

My relationship with migraine started about 15 years ago, a day like any other. I don't remember exactly how or when, because at that moment I didn't give it too much importance. I had had a headache for days, at the end of each day, and assumed it was from fatigue, until one day the pain became insufferable. The right side of my head hurt so badly that I couldn't even think. Everything bothered me: people, noise, lights... I was looking forward to getting home and going to bed. I did so and the pain passed, but it became more and more frequent. I decided to go to the doctor.

The Label

DIAGNOSIS: MIGRAINE. ACCORDING to the doctor, **I had to keep doing what I was already doing: taking a pain-killer and staying in a dark room, in silence, with nothing that could bother me**. I knew it well, as my mother had also suffered them.

I associated the first strong migraines with my menstruation. **The gynecologist told me it was normal, that**

it happened to a lot of women. She prescribed me anti-inflammatories. Later on, the story got complicated. The migraine began to appear after other triggers. The painkillers and anti-inflammatories did nothing to me and the intensity of the pain increased.

The Specialist (Genes, Triggers, Orderly Life)

I WAS REFERRED to a neurologist. After testing and confirming that it was a migraine, the doctor explained that **there was no cure and that it would probably get worse over time.** He also predicted that **my daughters would probably have it too, just as I had inherited it from my mother.**

He stressed the importance of finding the triggers to avoid them and, above all, to lead an orderly life: sleep eight hours, no alcohol, no dairy products, exercise, dark room whenever there are crises and a new medicine, specific and effective in tackling crises. That's how the triptans became part of my life.

I was an outstanding patient/student. I did everything by the book. The first few months were great. The neurologist's recommendations worked perfectly. Too bad the effect didn't last long. The days of pain were increasing, and I had to take between six and eight triptans a month. In addition, dizziness added to the migraine. The neurologist decided to try his luck with a new preventive treatment while I continued with the search for triggers and an orderly life.

The Alternatives

AT THE SAME time, as I saw that nothing was giving positive results, I started with the "alternatives": acupuncture, yoga, osteopathy, reiki, chiropractic, meditation, physiotherapy, piercing... they all promised me the cure or, at least, an improvement. But it seemed that I was the exception to the rule. Nothing took away my migraine or my dizziness.

Inheritance

AT THAT TIME, my oldest daughter, 15, started having migraines regularly. I couldn't believe it! She had them too, just like me and my mother. What bad luck! In fact, I had already been warned by the doctor... So, let's start with the protocol again: visit the neurologist, "migraine" label, painkillers and/or anti-inflammatories, dark room and orderly life. That last one was easy because at home, with me as a teacher, we were already doing it. So, the visits to the neurologist, the preventive medicines, the triptans, the days locked up in the dark in the room, were all multiplied by two.

Chronification

THE YEAR MY daughter started eleventh grade was the worst. We both had daily headaches, and three or four days a week the pain became an unbearable migraine. Even so, we always tried to live a normal life, to be strong and, as the professionals recommended, **"learn to live with it."** We visited more than one specialist, ear specialists, physiotherapists, osteopaths, psychologists, any professional who was recommended to us. All unsuccessfully. We finally decided to change neurologist, to look for the best specialist in migraines. It didn't matter what it cost or where we had to move. And we found her. With all our hopes pinned on her, we both went to her office. That day was one of the worst days of our lives. She confirmed something we already knew, that **migraine was an incurable disease. She said that our brain was hyperexcitable** and that's why everything bothered it. Worst of all, it was a mysterious disease. What was really going on was not well known, despite all the research.

Living in the Cave

SO THE ONLY solution was to lead a practically unleadable life: to sleep just 8 hours, no more and no less, to get up every day at the same time, to exercise, "but neither too much nor too little," not to expose ourselves directly to the light, "to live like in a cave," to rest whenever we needed it and to be in darkness during crises. Make a list of triggers and avoid them all: sun, chocolate, sushi, alcohol, going out at night, going to the movies, taking a nap and so on. Oh! And take preventive medication, plus anti-inflammatories and triptans.

Despair

MY DAUGHTER COLLAPSED. She was in pain every day and so much medication left her groggy, making the effort to study insufferable. When we no longer saw a solution or a way out of the situation, the doctor told us that there was a novel treatment, botox, which was working well. That maybe we could try it... were we going to say no to the only way out that we could see in that hell of a life?

From that visit on and the next two, with botox included, everything got worse. Every morning I woke up with a migraine and the first thing I had to do was take a triptan. I started having migraines with all the triggers that the doctor had mentioned, which confirmed that I was a migraine expert and that I was right. So, I had to follow everything she said. My daughter was taking all the prescribed medication, even when it left her very groggy. She kept studying everything she could and more to get the grades she needed. We ended up in the emergency room twice in a week: my daughter couldn't stand the pain and needed more painkillers. They did scans and tests again and, as expected, everything went well. We went back to the neurologist. My daughter told her that the medicines didn't do anything. The last thing the neurologist said was that it was impossible, that **she couldn't possibly have so much pain. That with medication we should be able to live a normal life**.

It was obvious that she had not seen her crying in pain day after day, in the dark in her room, missing everything that life has to offer a teenager... That was our last visit to the neurologist, now two years ago.

Defenselessness

MY DAUGHTER FINISHED the school year exhausted, but with brilliant grades. The day it ended, in tears, she told me that **she would not take any more medication and**

that she wanted to stop studying. She couldn't bear to go on living with so much suffering.

The feeling of despair was insufferable, and that same day, like so many others throughout ten years, I stood in front of the computer ready to find another treatment, another "better neurologist." I wasn't going to give up. There had to be something. And the name of Dr. Arturo Goicoechea appeared. I started reading his blog and was amazed. How could I not have heard of him before? Everything he said made so much sense. From that day on, our life turned a hundred and eighty degrees. I got his book "Migraine. A brain nightmare." and, as I read it, many ideas began to fit in my head. Actually, the way we had managed our migraine wasn't the right one. Neurobiology had the answer to many of my doubts. Thus, I decided to leave behind everything I had learned until then and start over.

2 LEAVING THE CAVE

We have heard Montse's story many times from the patients that attend our courses. Before trying Education on Biology, they had tried all the offers of the flea market of official and alternative remedies. They are castaways...

THE VERDICT OF Neurology is conclusive: **you suffer from a genetic brain disease, mysterious, irreversible. In your case, difficult to control and, from what it seems, you have transmitted it to your kids.**

After trying everything without success, Montse ended up on the Internet. There, she found more of the same: the official explanations and the alternatives, all the therapies they promised. Perhaps they seemed to be working at first, but then they abandoned her, unable to neutralize that damned genetic condition of her brain, which had gained strength over time.

She finally found something different:

Know pain, no pain. Know migraine, no migraine. Hm, let's see…

It talked about the brain, neurons, learning… about courses for patients… about errors in assessing the threat to the organism… of the Neuroimmune System… At least it seemed different from what she had read and heard so far.

Pain is something that requires an explanation[1]. You may have to understand, know, what's going on in your head. When we understand something, we stop fearing it, said Marie Curie.

I welcome you to this book. I'll try to explain the biological plot of the migraine. Forget about your condition as a patient in search of a solution.

You're a student. You want to know what's actually going on in your head.

You've been a good student, too. That's why you learned, like Montse, to suffer from migraine. Keep being that good student. We need her. Maybe the problem is in the books used, in the teachers. Perhaps you have inherited and passed on the genes of excellence as a student to your daughters.

Forget about migraine and get interested in Biology, in the human organism.

---

[1] Anne Carson. *Plainwater: Essays and Poetry.*; 2000

3 WHAT IS A MIGRAINE?

He had never cared too much about what exactly migraine was. What he needed was an effective treatment. A mysterious and irreversible disease, they told him. All the therapies he tried had been useless. Maybe, he thought for himself, he was suffering a particularly severe form of migraine, resistant to therapies.
Maybe not.

YOU DON'T NEED me to explain what a migraine crisis feels like. If you have it, you know it perfectly well:

An intense pain, sometimes "throbbing" (later I will clarify the reason for the quotation marks), maybe only appearing in one half of the head, and always accompanied by nausea, vomiting and intolerance to sensory stimuli (lights, sounds, smells).

What may be happening inside the head becomes unthinkable. There are those who imagine very dilated arteries, inflamed and struck by a violent heartbeat. Others think of increased pressure inside the skull. Most people end up giving up imagining what is happening and just want the torture to end, although they suspect it will come back at its convenience.

Actually, nothing really happens in the head. Arteries are normal. No dilation, no inflammation. The pressure inside the head is also normal. That's the problem. Normalcy. The mystery. There's nothing worse than not knowing what is going on, because, obviously, something is going on. Pain, vomiting, sensory intolerance are real.

How can everything be normal?

Sometimes a migraine crisis is "triggered" by something known, although you almost never know why. The head may be a complicated, sensitive place, subject to the stress of modern life, the noises, the lights, the hustle and bustle of the city. That's what you've been made to understand. Don't believe it.

Our organism is sufficiently adapted to manage stressful scenarios. Neurons do not smoke or generate toxic molecules when mental hustle and bustle increases. If the circuits and connections are "heated," a *synaptic scaling* mechanism is activated[2] that lowers the "temperature"; the heart supports physical, cardiac-healthy activity; the lungs have no problem getting the necessary air; the

---

[2] Fernandes D, Carvalho AL. Mechanisms of homeostatic plasticity in the excitatory synapse. *J Neurochem*. 2016. doi:10.1111/jnc.13687

kidneys filter blood; the liver metabolizes whatever arrives from the intestine. There is healthy activity in all the neighborhoods and guilds of the organism. The brain has fun accompanying the individual, the game of life, the exploration.

It's hard to believe that the head is normal, but it is. If it were opened in the middle of a crisis, we wouldn't find any anomaly. Don't waste any more time with your guesses. Your head, outside and inside, is normal.

It's a matter of the brain. It's also normal, but it acts in a way, say, strange, wrong. Ramachandran, a famous neuroscientist, says that pain is **an opinion**[3]. Yes. Sounds strange. You'll have to get used to hearing strange claims about the brain.

A migraine is the consequence of an erroneous cerebral opinion, of which you are not aware, but it is in your best interest to be so. The brain shouldn't opine-act that way. It has no justification and provides nothing but mortification and disability. Don't let the security of your body be managed by a mistaken brain.

They may have explained to you that migraine is written in the genes. If there were more cases in your family, it would seem reasonable... and disheartening. You saw

---

[3] Ramachandran VS, Bakeslee S, Sacks O. Phantoms in the Brain: Probing the Mysteries of the Human Mind.; 1999.

your mother suffer, anticipating what is now your turn, because of those genes inherited from her.

Except in extremely rare cases, there are no genes that produce migraine. There may be genes that increase the likelihood of crises, but the universe of gene expression is more complex than it seems. A gene is involved in many factors and each factor is influenced by multiple genes. The genome contains the recipes of the kitchen of life, but from recipe to dish (the expression of those recipes) there is a complex path. They say that the zip code (where one is born and raised) is more important than the genetic code (from whom one is born).

Okay. Let me uncover my proposal:

Migraines are not a genetic brain disease. There's no mystery in their guts and they can be deactivated. Migraines are learned.

Nature versus nurture.

It's something that is cooked when learning, in a normal brain. The brain manages the organism, but it does so from an idea, a story, built on that organism, as it interacts with the environment. That story is the most important biological function. You, the conscious individual, will reside in it and will suffer the consequences that derive from it.

Forget about genes, the orderly life, what you eat, what you sleep or don't sleep, stress, time or hormonal changes, your arteries, your neck, your postures when using a computer.

The brain doesn't have a bin to get rid of it all, but it does have a storage room. Let all that migraine culture go to the storage room and try not to visit it, letting go of the temptation that there might be something there worth rescuing. Don't fall into Diogenes syndrome either, accumulating everything you hear and believe, by inability to get rid of it.

Maybe, your relatives' migraines contributed to facilitating by imitation, by fear, the "migraineous learning." Maybe, there were no previous records in your case. They are not necessary. The culture is there. The brain absorbs its contents without asking for permission. Learning is basically unconscious. You will know what your brain has learned when the story it builds (behind your back) becomes conscious and expresses itself for the first time as a crisis, your first crisis. That is the key moment, the day when the story comes out to the screen of consciousness, to you. It is the moment of questions, uncertainty, fears, consultations with experts, alertness, therapies ...

Once the pilgrimage to the remedy flea market is complete, it is time to check whether the story your brain has built over the years should be thwarted.

Migraine is not transmitted through genes. It is transmitted through the expert culture. Bring the migraine culture to the storage room. It's time for biology. Migraine is a story, a narrative.

If migraine can be learned, it can, perhaps, be unlearned. Give yourself a chance.

Know pain, no pain. Know migraine, no migraine.

4 THE BRAIN IS NOT INFALLIBLE.

You have nothing to lose, but your pain
(Kevin Allcoat).
An English reader of my blog wrote this comment.
Knowledge has a place in the connectivity of the complex neural network. Beliefs and expectations impose their law in the decisions of the brain, in the states of the organism.

I'M NOT GOING to give you solutions. Don't be frustrated by it. I will try to transmit to you a tool, more powerful than any therapy: **the knowledge of what is really happening**[4].

What I'm about to explain to you will not be politically correct. It will probably be the first time you hear about it. You have heard, read and believed just the opposite,

---

[4] Mittinty MM, Vanlint S, Stocks N, Mittinty MN, Moseley GL. Exploring effect of pain education on chronic pain patients' expectation of recovery and pain intensity. *Scand J Pain*. 2018. doi:10.1515/sjpain-2018-0023

but I assure you that all these concepts are biologically correct, adjusted to what, most certainly, we know about the organism. At best, politically correct information is biologically incomplete, and even incorrect.

It is hard to believe that all this torture can go away **"just talking" (or reading)**, when the most expensive and powerful drugs, prescribed by the most renowned professionals, alternative therapies, diets, the boring orderly life, all the imaginable deprivations have not succeeded... I assure you that, even if you were not aware of it, they have talked to your brain about organism matters, about headaches, for example. Maybe you acquired migraines unconsciously, **"just talking,"** just observing and imitating[5]. Don't underestimate learning. Do not limit it to the language.

In recent decades, much progress has been made in understanding biological processes, especially neurons, their circuits, how they acquire and process information. Probably nobody has talked to you about it, but they have kept telling you about other things: genes, hormones, stress, food.

There is nothing in the body that is not managed by the Nervous System, a complex network of neurons that

---

[5] Richter M, Eck J, Straube T, Miltner WHR, Weiss T. Do words hurt? Brain activation during the processing of pain-related words. *Pain*. 2010. doi:10.1016/j.pain.2009.08.009

evaluate everything, relentlessly, and "make decisions" based on those evaluations.

Everything we feel, think and do, emotions, pain, nausea, the need to isolate ourselves, all of this arises from the activity of neurons. If they put electrodes on our heads, they'll register a complex pattern of electrical potentials, an *electroencephalogram*. These patterns reflect in each moment what the brain is "saying," proposing and deciding on all kinds of issues, the external and internal world, the past, present and future.

Evidently the "opinion" of the brain is absurd in this case. There is no situation that justifies the crisis. It doesn't have any benefit. Quite the opposite. We could interpret that situation as a mistake.

It is hard to believe that all the barbarity of migraines is the consequence of an evaluative error, of a mistaken cerebral opinion. It is easier to accept that something abnormal, sick, produces all these symptoms. It is essential that you are aware of the existence of this complex network dedicated to updating beliefs and expectations. You may need to see it to believe it, but you need to believe it (understand it) to see it.

That which for us is so simple, like being a certain *I* who feels, thinks, decides, suffers, is motivated and demotivated, has its ups and downs... is the mirror of that continuous unconscious evaluative activity of our neural network. It weaves and unweaves the story of the organism it must watch over and protect. But don't be over-confident. The brain is not perfect, omnipotent or infallible. Quite the opposite.

You may think it's idiotic, but... the brain is an idiot[6].

---

[6] Burnett D. The Idiot Brain: A Neuroscientist Explains the Imperfections of Our Gray Matter; 2016.

5 THE BRAIN, AN EXPENSIVE AND RISKY INVESTMENT

At least, it's surprising. It's not a sick brain, it's an idiot brain. It may make sense. The lungs, the heart, the kidneys, are healthy or sick, but they are not wrong. There's no room for idiocy in them. But the brain... perhaps yes, it is an idiot or, simply, obedient, tamable, incautious, ignorant...

OUR SPECIES (HOMO sapiens, ma non troppo) evolved towards an increase in the size and complexity of the brain. The current one weighs about 1.5 kg, i.e. 2% of body weight. However, it consumes 20% of the energy[7]. It's very expensive. Was it really worth it, from what we're seeing? Is the cost/benefit ratio profitable?

From the point of view of survival and reproductive success, it is apparent that it was a success. From a welfare

---

[7] Raichle ME, Gusnard DA. Appraising the brain's energy budget. *Proc Natl Acad Sci U S A*. 2002. doi:10.1073/pnas.17239949

point of view, it's not so clear. We are probably the most distressed, neurotic, depressed and aching species on the planet. The human brain is very good at ensuring our survival, but it has many side effects.

What does the brain spend all that energy on? First of all, the expense is practically constant, whether we are in the middle of a mental hustle and bustle or if we are navel-gazing or daydreaming. It is always activated, using 100% of its capacity.

There is no clear explanation for this fixed expense. A plausible proposal suggests that the network is constantly thought of and updated, keeping something for us as simple as the "I," the awareness of existing, of being on each scenario. One's consciousness demands a great deal of brain activity. Otherwise it would fade away.

When the brain is liberated from the requests of the conscious individual, it attends to its tasks, which include organizing all the activity of being in the world, in each of the scenarios, evaluating the costs and benefits for the organism, which derive from the behavior of the individual. We're a species with an especially ruminant mind.

Are we *sapiens* really so sapiens? Does all that constant brain activity generate intelligence, correct evaluations, common sense? Migraines aren't exactly a sign of intelligent brain behavior. The brain panics without anything that's threatening the head. It does it over and over again, with increasing intensity. It does not change with therapies, with pharmacological containment, with relaxation, strict diets...

The question is: are we already born with that dangerous drift toward absurd alarmist "opinions" or does the brain construct, assimilate an unintelligent theory of the organism it is supposed to protect?

Do genes determine this aberrant behavior or has learning generated this uncontrollable panic, which triggers the alarm without any justification?[8]

Is it a hardware problem or software problem?

Are we born programmed or can we program ourselves? Are we programmed in learning and can we deprogram ourselves?

---

[8] Colloca L. Nocebo effects can make you feel pain. *Science (80-)*. 2017. doi:10.1126/science.aap8488

6 SYMPTOMS

Continuous evaluative flow; we are ruminant beings; it has not been a good idea to bet on mental guts; the brain has become "migrained."
Programs. Maybe the culture of the organism is the one that controls that programming and is a bad travel companion.

THERE IS AN important biological function that few speak of: the **assessment function** of the risk, costs, benefits, uncertainties, which contains each action, each scenario. Symptoms express what your brain is saying at that moment, place and circumstance, based on the information acquired throughout your life.

MIGRAINE = LABEL

"MIGRAINE" IS JUST a label. It comes from the phonetic degradation of the Greek *hemi-kranea* (half head) and highlights that odd condition of pain, often affecting only one half of the head. *He-micrania* led to *micrania*-migraine. We tend to fall into the illusion that by naming things we begin to control them (nominal fallacy). Don't get caught up in a word. It's just a wrapper. The important thing here is the content.

MIGRAINE = STATE OF ALERTNESS-PROTECTION

A CRISIS IS the consequence of the evaluative state of that moment. In the language of the organism it is a **state of alertness-protection**. The crisis doesn't start with pain. When you pre-feel it you are already in it, in the alertness state of your organism. It would be nice if you didn't get caught up in that state, but it's not easy[9].

In some cases, in approximately 20% of patients, the alertness state generates worrisome but harmless symptoms, such as loss of vision on one side of the visual field, inability to speak, or tingling on one side of the body. Neurologists call it "aura."

The visual processing areas are activated and enter a loop of increasing hyperactivity, which surpasses the ability of neurons to generate an electrical signal. It would be

---

[9] Dodick DW. A Phase-by-Phase Review of Migraine Pathophysiology. *Headache*. 2018. doi:10.1111/head.13300

a metabolic exhaustion, an exhaustion of the battery. We have to wait for it to load again. It has nothing to do with circulation.

Sometimes the crisis ends there: the unrest and the aura. You regain vision, sensation, or language and go back to normal. It would be a migraine without pain or vomiting. More often, the aura is followed by the typical crisis (pain, vomiting, and sensory intolerance). This means that, in addition to the state of alertness, the organism has activated protection resources. It has gone from guarding to protecting.

Most commonly, the crisis is initiated by a state of alertness (prodromes) that does not generate the aura and that leads to the state of active protection, pain, vomiting and sensory intolerance.

I advise you to eliminate the label "migraine" and internalize "unjustified state of alertness-protection" every time the crisis occurs[10].

In children, protection often focuses on the abdomen or a limb. "Abdominal migraine" or "migraine of an arm or leg." As they become an adult, the pain leaves their

---

[10] Charles A. Migraine: a brain state. *Curr Opin Neurol.* 2013. doi:10.1097/WCO.0b013e32836085f4

guts or limbs and settles on their head (on half of it, sometimes)[11].

It seems, therefore, that it is not, in origin at least, a specific problem of the head. The brain guards-protects different areas, depending on age. Sometimes it does not substitute one place for another, but adds up and ends up consolidating the generalized pain. The labels appear: "irritable colon," "fibromyalgia," "chronic pain," "low back pain," "cervical pain". The state of alertness-protection is expressed in many places and in different ways. We could talk about "lumbar migraine," "cervical migraine," "vestibular migraine." Even that state can lead to cervical stiffness in children.

A label doesn't tell you what's going on. Heed the advice. Remove the label, the stigma. Think about what is really going on: an **"evaluative error of my organism,"** a **false alarm.**

You must know with absolute conviction that your head is in no danger. As much as the siren sounds and the police, firefighters and ambulances have come over and over again, you have to get the certainty that it is an absurd, disturbing, insufferable deployment. Your house

---

[11] Gelfand AA. Migraine and childhood periodic syndromes in children and adolescents. *Curr Opin Neurol.* 2013. doi:10.1097/WCO.0b013e32836085c7

is not going to fall down, it will not burn down, nobody is coming in to rob you.

Let's talk about the Neuroimmune System. It is the one who builds that absurd story that makes you a martyr.

7 THE NEUROIMMUNE SYSTEM

Every time I write Neuroimmune, the Word proofreader under-
lines it in red. It's an unrecognized term.
The Immune System is the one that puts on the medals of defensive
successes and bears the blush of errors when it protects us from
harmless agents. Allergic and anaphylactic reactions are the con-
sequence of seeing danger where there is none.
However, neurons are of paramount importance in defensive
work.
Let us do them justice, to praise them or condemn them.

THE ORGANISM IS BEING WATCHED AND DEFENDED

THERE ARE EXTERNAL and internal threats that must be detected to avoid damage. A migraine crisis corresponds to the activation of a state of emergency, due to the assessment by "the defenses" that the head is in danger. You're not the one making that assessment. You don't even know that there is this function of valuing, evaluating danger.

We have a vague idea of "defenses," antibodies and things like that. The organism has the resources to detect threats of all kinds and implement the corresponding protection responses.

We have been told about the Immune System, a network of mobile cells that patrol the body and detect the presence of germs and cancer cells. Surprisingly and unfairly, we have not been told anything about the defensive Nervous System, a network of neurons organized in circuits, each in its place, immobile. At its care, the detection of physical and chemical states that may alter the physical integrity of tissues.

In fact, when we speak of "defenses," we should always refer to the **Neuroimmune System**, and consider both subsystems: the one formed by the cells of the Immune System and the complex network of neuronal circuits that also watches and protects us. They work absolutely integrated, with a common language[12] [13].

---

[12] Pinho-Ribeiro FA, Verri WA, Chiu IM. Nociceptor Sensory Neuron–Immune Interactions in Pain and Inflammation. *Trends Immunol.* 2017. doi:10.1016/j.it.2016.10.001

[13] Grace PM, Hutchinson MR, Maier SF, Watkins LR. Pathological pain and the neuroimmune interface. *Nat Rev Immunol.* 2014. doi:10.1038/nri3621

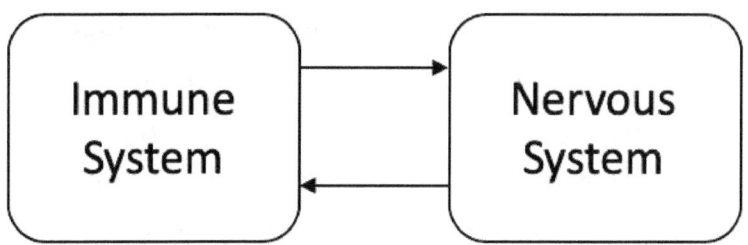

Each subsystem is responsible for detecting different threats. The immune subsystem deals with biological threats (germs, cancer) and the neuronal subsystem, in addition, with the physical-chemical ones: extreme temperatures, compressions, stretching, acids, lack of blood supply.

CONGENITAL NEUROIMMUNE COMPONENT

AT BIRTH, WE already have detection and response resources for many biological and physicochemical threats. They have been selected throughout evolution and appear in the genome. They make up the **congenital neuroimmune component.** Thanks to it, we detect the presence of bacteria, viruses, fungi and parasites (Immune subsystem) or thermal, mechanical and harmful chemical stimuli (neuronal subsystem). Congenital component evaluations are always accurate. They have passed the filter of evolution. They have proven their reliability after millions of years of experience.

However, the congenital Neuroimmune catalogue of the dangerous is not complete. There are biological and physicochemical variables that may correspond to agents and threatening states that are not registered in the congenital component, and the Neuroimmune System must classify them as danger reporters.

ACQUIRED COMPONENT

WE WILL HAVE measles, but only once. The **acquired component** will have incorporated the registration of the molecules that identify the virus and will activate the defensive resources quickly in another contagion.

The congenital component is infallible, but the acquired one can be wrong and is wrong in many cases. Sometimes it doesn't detect the threat (**false negative**) and other times it sees danger where there isn't (**false positive**). It learns from error-trial-error... but only if it detects and corrects that error as such.

Cancer is the consequence of the error of inability to see threat in a colony of cells that have managed to circumvent the Neuroimmune surveillance (false negative). Unidentified danger. Allergy and migraines are the consequence of evaluating as danger, even if there is no danger (false positive)[14]. False alarm.

The acquired Neuroimmune component **imagines** (fears) damage, anticipates it, predicts it, and acts on that evaluation. It can make a mistake and it can detect the error and correct it, but that's not always the case. It makes the same mistake over and over again.

Errors due to false positives of the Neuroimmune System make up an extensive section of Pathology: **autoneuroimmune diseases, or diseases due to unnecessary overprotection.**

MIGRAINE = AUTONEUROIMMUNE DISEASE

MIGRAINES ARE AN autoneuroimmune disease, the consequence of a threat assessment error by the defensive neuronal network. It is caused by the organism, its defensive neuronal subsystem, which evaluates, in this case, threats when and where there is none. The individual is limited to suffering the consequences and seeking help from professionals. It seems complicated, but try to see the simple logic. What's new is always complicated, especially if it's contrary to what you have learned and automated.

---

[14] Mehle ME. Migraine and allergy: A review and clinical update. *Curr Allergy Asthma Rep.* 2012. doi:10.1007/s11882-012-0251-x

Reflect for a moment on this fundamental idea:

Allergies and autoimmune diseases arise in a reasonably healthy organism as a result of a <u>threat assessment error</u> by the Immune System. This is a well-known, acceptable statement. Politically correct. Migraines and other labels such as fibromyalgia, chronic pain, arise in a reasonably healthy organism as a result of a <u>threat assessment error</u> by the defensive neural network. It sounds strange, novel, unknown, but it is simple, once understood and accepted. It is alleviating to know that it is not the victim who is responsible but the network of neurons, the neuronal subsystem of the Neuroimmune System.

8 ORGANISM CULTURE

Geneticist Theodosius Dobzhansky coined the phrase: "nothing in biology makes sense except in the light of evolution."

We could nuance the statement by referring to human biology, highlighting the importance of culture, the information that experts accumulate, with successes and errors, about the organism.

In order to understand the biology of migraines, given that it is an exclusive condition of the human species, we must consider what differentiates us from other species, the complexity of our brain, its imaginative-predictive capacity.

Reflecting on the Biology of migraines forces us to consider the role of culture, the interpretation that experts make of the label "migraine."

MIGRAINE AND OTHER similar labels, jointly considered as "symptoms without medical explanation," express, as I propose, a threat assessment error by the Neuroimmune System. I remind you that having a label called "migraine" does not explain anything.

EVOLUTIONARY SENSE OF HEADACHE

THIS STATE OF **unjustified alertness-protection** is expressed in consciousness as pain, nauseous sensation and sensory intolerance. What is the evolutionary sense of headaches? What is their benefit?

Don't use what you have been told. Don't think about genes, stress, food, weather changes, and hormonal changes. That's culture, indoctrination. We had brought all that to the storage room. Try to think in a biological, evolutionary way. What would you have to do to cause yourself pain right now in a part of your body?

You can do many things: pinch yourself, pull your hair, bring your hand close to a hot spot, take an ice cube, make a tight tourniquet in your arm ... that is, **damage** yourself. Doing something that can violently destroy tissue: applying mechanical energy (tearing, compressing), thermal energy (heat, cold) or chemical energy (preventing the arrival of blood). The pain would inform you of the damage caused or the imminent danger of damage, if you do not avoid the dangerous stimulus, and would force you to get rid of it.

The pain **informs** the conscious individual and **protects a threatened area.** Do you believe that in a migraine crisis there is such a threatening situation?

I can assure you, there isn't. The organism acts, without knowing it, on the basis of an erroneous evaluation. No trigger contains a real threat of violent destruction of the head. Thus, the state of alertness-protection shouldn't have to be activated.

NAUSEA

WHAT BIOLOGICAL SENSE do you see in nausea? When does it make sense to perform a stomach pump? Logically, when one suspects that one has taken a jar of pills, when one assesses that there is a harmful agent that has entered through the digestive tract.

When the Neuroimmune System sees a threat projected over the inside, it activates the vomiting resource. It does not do so when the threat is in the entrance (mouth) or in the locomotor apparatus. Trigeminal neuralgia, cluster headache, a toothache, an acute herniated disc, are accompanied by intense pain, but without vomiting, as the threat does not refer to the visceral interior[15].

---

[15] Maniyar FH, Sprenger T, Schankin C, Goadsby PJ. The origin of nausea in migraine–A PET study. *J Headache Pain*. 2014. doi:10.1186/1129-2377-15-84

SENSORY INTOLERANCE

WHAT ABOUT INTOLERANCE to stimuli (lights, sounds, smells...)? In the same line of thinking in evolutionary terms, the organism forces you to stay in the den, in a protected place, without stimuli. Anything that involves a threatening exterior is unbearable. The more you feel like living a normal life, the greater the intolerance, the unbearability of the stimuli. Migraine patients try to continue their normal life, go to work, to dinner organized by friends, but their organism makes it difficult, heroic.

The need to look for an explanation and a possible solution leads us to consider those proposals contained in culture. We think about genes, arteries, food, changes in weather, hormones, that is, topics that the expert information provides. However, they do not teach us to reflect on the real biological causes, the biological and physico-chemical states and agents capable of violently destroying tissues.

Nor do they inform us of the risk of error in the defensive neural network, as is the case with its Immune equivalent. Don't search yourself. Biologically search your organism, your Neuroimmune System. The only biologically justified and explained triggers of pain would be states and agents that violently destroy our cells.

9 CORRELATION DOES NOT IMPLY CAUSATION

The Neuroimmune System is not infallible. In its eagerness to find the states and agents capable of generating unexpected, violent cell death, it sometimes blames what it shouldn't blame-and rushes to its conclusions. Paying for the sins of others.
Migraines are like allergies. The organism overprotects itself. The individual doesn't matter.

FIRST OF ALL, an important warning: do not confuse correlation with causation.

We tend to conclude hastily that, if an event B follows a previous one A, it means that A has caused B. If I have eaten chocolate or there is south wind, and then I have a migraine crisis, it's because the chocolate or the south wind caused the migraine. If I take an ibuprofen and then the pain is gone, it is because the ibuprofen has removed the pain.

It seems reasonable, but don't trust appearances. The continuous evaluation process always looks for all possible correlations between events, and when a possible one appears, in the absence of a better one, it stays with it, as if it were a definitive explanation. Don't settle for that. Psychologists talk about *causal illusion.*

If B follows A, A may have caused B. Maybe, but it's not always like that. You'll never be wrong if you use this other conclusion about pain:

If the correlation of having a crisis after eating chocolate really exists, you may conclude that the body evaluates the action of eating chocolate as dangerous to your head, as if a state of violent tissue destruction were to occur (for example, a meningeal infection or a hemorrhage). It is absurd, but that would be the correct interpretation from the biological, evolutionary point of view.

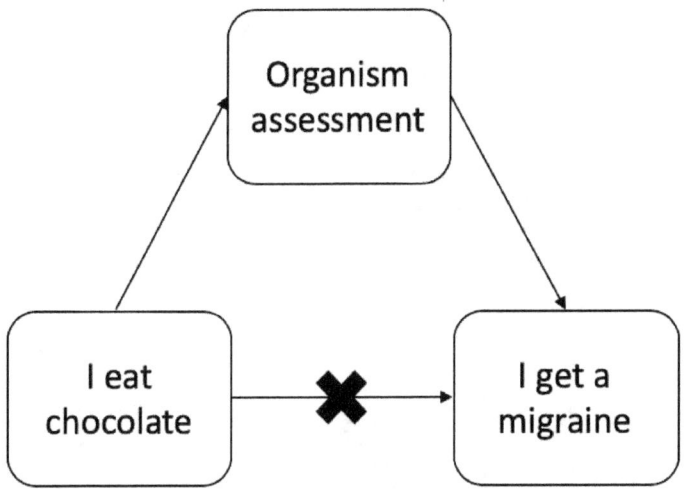

I know. It's hard to believe, or at least it sounds weird, complicated.

I give you the example of the Immune System with allergies: if you breathe air with pollen, sneeze and your eyes water, it is not because of pollen, but because of the erroneous evaluation made by your Immune System, which acts **as if** pollen were something dangerous, a germ.

If the air did not contain pollen, sneezes would not happen, but pollen is not the **cause.** It's the wrong evaluation of the Immune System.

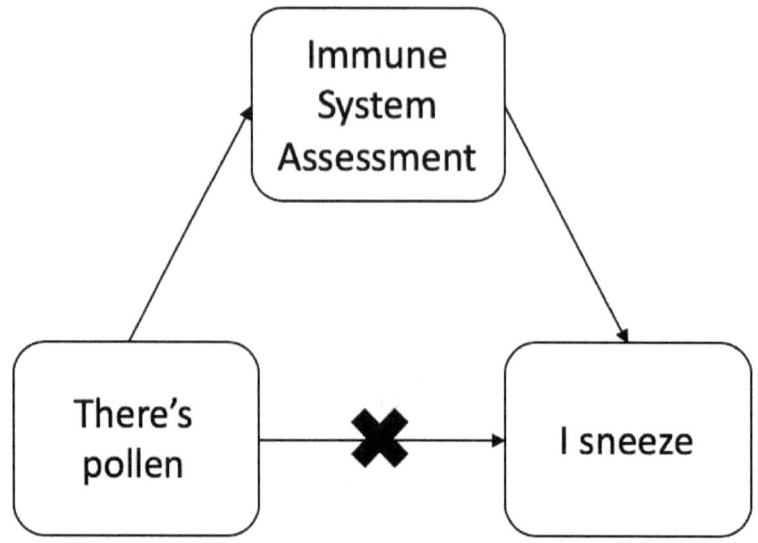

"In my experience." Three dangerous words in all sorts of matters. Don't cling to your checks of whether A, then B.

10 WHERE DOES PAIN COME FROM?

Conscience is deceptive. The brain is not looking for truth but for survival. The contents of the conscious screen often reflect what the brain fears.
The fear of unprogrammed cell death becomes pain, projected into the space occupied by the skull, the abdomen or a foot. It looks like that pain occurs where we feel it as a result, necessarily, of some disturbance.

IF I TWIST my foot and a sprain occurs, I will feel pain in the foot, but does the feeling of pain really occur in the foot? That is what it seems from "your experience" and because there is a correlation, but the correct answer is more complicated.

To establish the origin of the pain, researchers apply harmful stimuli to various tissues. That's the way they do it in the head. They find that by stimulating the meninges (membranes covering the brain and spinal cord), the great vessels (arteries and veins), and the trigeminal nerve terminals (responsible for collecting information on everything that happens inside the skull), a feeling of pain is produced. These tissues are sensitive to harmful stimuli.

However, if the brain is stimulated, none of the points cause pain. It is possible to intervene in the brain without applying general anesthesia, with the patient being awake, without feeling pain. "The brain doesn't hurt," it was said, and it's still said.

The fact is that researchers focus their studies on the tissues that do generate the feeling of pain when stimulated[16] [17]. Initially, they thought the pain was in the great vessels (arteries and veins). Migraines, it was concluded, were a vascular pain. It may sound familiar: arteries contract first, and that causes little blood to reach certain areas of the brain. It was thought that lack of blood supply would explain the aura. After the contraction, an intense dilation would come as a reaction, and that dilation would explain the pain.

---

[16] Burgos-Vega C, Moy J, Dussor G. Meningeal afferent signaling and the pathophysiology of migraine. In: *Progress in Molecular Biology and Translational Science.* ; 2015. doi:10.1016/bs.pmbts.2015.01.001

[17] Goadsby PJ, Holland PR, Martins-Oliveira M, Hoffmann J, Schankin C, Akerman S. Pathophysiology of Migraine: A Disorder of Sensory Processing. *Physiol Rev.* 2017. doi:10.1152/physrev.00034.2015

That was said and continues to be said on the Internet and in many consultations. Dilated, swollen arteries that cause pain with each heartbeat. However, current imaging technology makes it possible to see the arteries in the course of a crisis, to measure their caliber, the amount of blood circulating. Now we know they're not dilated[18]. The vascular theory is dead.

Only the trigeminal nerve terminals, distributed by the meninges and the great vessels, remained as suspicious tissue. The pain would arise from those trigemino-vascular terminals. The vascular theory was dead. The *trigemino-vascular theory* for the origin of pain was born.

Suppose those trigeminal nerve terminals are the source of the pain. If something pathological were to happen in those meninges, such as an infection, a hemorrhage, a necrosis event, it is logical and desirable that pain should appear after the sensitization of those terminals by the dead and inflamed tissues. But nothing happens during a migraine crisis. There is no necrosis or inflammation that sensitizes the trigeminal. Thus, if the head hurts, it is only possible, they say, if those terminals are sensitized by another mechanism.

---

[18] Schoonman GG, Van Der Grond J, Kortmann C, Van Der Geest RJ, Terwindt GM, Ferrari MD. Migraine headache is not associated with cerebral or meningeal vasodilatation - A 3T magnetic resonance angiography study. *Brain*. 2008. doi:10.1093/brain/awn094

In recent decades, techniques have been developed that allow us to visualize brain activity. Applying these novel neuroimaging techniques, it has been seen that, in the course of a migraine crisis, certain brain areas are activated. That makes one think the crisis originates in them. They've called them "migraine generators[19]."

The brain does not hurt, (one starts from that premise) when stimulated, but the genetic migraine condition can create those hyperexcitable "generators" that, without anything threatening happening, produce the trigeminal sensitization, a necessary condition (it is said) for the individual to feel pain. They say.

The brain gets excited and this excitation ends up sensitizing the trigeminal vasculomeningeal terminals, generating pain with any stimulus (arterial beats, a small movement), even if nothing threatening happens (infection, hemorrhage). They say.

The key is in that supposed "generator" with which every migraine (it is said) is born. The triggers would be external stimuli of all kinds or internal variables, which would ignite those easily excitable generators. The patients with that generator would be, perhaps, perfectionists, sensitive people or perhaps the rhythm of life, stress,

---

[19] Schulte LH, May A. Of generators, networks and migraine attacks. *Curr Opin Neurol.* 2017. doi:10.1097/WCO.0000000000000441

hormonal changes... would facilitate their triggers. They say.

That is what the current official doctrine suggests. Genes, lifestyle, emotional tensions, excesses and defects of all kinds. The genetically sensitive generator would jump easily. The official theory may, at least, be questionable. I'll explain later.

In many cases, in addition to the pain with migraine pedigree (half head, vomiting, sensory intolerance), there is headache without these characteristics. Neurologists talk about *tension headache*. The muscles of the neck, of the jaw, would be stiff, from stress, nervous tension. They say.

The genes explain migraines, and the stress and muscle contracture that it supposedly generates, the "tension headache." The responsible one: the individual. He doesn't manage his life well. He doesn't relax. He's not sitting properly. He's twitching, he's contracted. They say.

Perfectionist personality? What's wrong with that. I would like to always be attended to by perfectionists: the car mechanic, the plumber...

11 HOWEVER

The expert culture of migraines has been evolving. Enraged gods, unbalanced moods, dilated and swollen arteries, "generator" genes, unproductive stress, stiff muscles, excessive CGRP, sensitive ion channels.
Culture, at the moment, does not question itself. What everyone preaches is not questionable. There's cake for all the proposals. You have to try them all to stay with the one that works. The truth is not in the truth, but in the benefit that each person obtains.
It's working!
That'll do.

THE BRAIN DOES HURT

IT'S NOT TRUE that the brain doesn't hurt. There are areas (the posterior insula and the medial operculum) which, if stimulated, cause the feeling of "pain" in consciousness. The neurosurgeon Wilder Penfield described the maps of representation of the body in the brain, stimulating the cortex point by point, and pointed out that none of them evoked pain[20], but he did not stimulate punctually the zone that does hurt when stimulated.

THE PAIN NEUROMATRIX

THAT ZONE IS the one that receives the information of the damaged or threatened tissues and then sends it to an extensive network of areas, distributed by the cerebral cortex, the "Pain Neuromatrix," the neural network that produces it when it is activated.

Pain does not arise from the stimulation of the initial reception area, but from the fact that stimulation activates the processing network. Only then does the feeling of "pain" appear.

On the other hand, if he had **simultaneously** stimulated all areas of the "pain neuromatrix" he would also have evoked pain. If you have to enter a password and try each of the numbers separately, you will get nothing. You have to enter them all at once. The key to pain lies in the simultaneous activation of that "Neuromatrix."

So, the brain does hurt. It's the only one who can generate any perception. For example, pain.

---

[20] PENFIELD W, BOLDREY E. SOMATIC MOTOR AND SENSORY REPRESENTATION IN THE CEREBRAL CORTEX OF MAN AS STUDIED BY ELECTRICAL STIMULATION. *Brain*. 1937. doi:10.1093/brain/60.4.389

Headache Doesn't Beat

On the other hand, and I clarify the quotation marks, pain does not "beat". The rhythm of the feeling of pain, the hammering that is sometimes felt and interpreted as the impact of the heartbeat on a swollen, dilated artery, does not come from the artery. The frequency of the heartbeat does not match that of the pain. It doesn't change with activity and rest. What gives it its rhythmic character is the electrical activity of central brain oscillators. Nothing to do with the arteries, but with the electrical support of the evaluative flow of that moment[21] [22].

Incomprehensibly, experts continue to refer to migraine pain as throbbing (without quotation marks).

---

[21] Mo J, Maizels M, Ding M, Ahn AH. Does throbbing pain have a brain signature? *Pain*. 2013. doi:10.1016/j.pain.2013.02.013

[22] Mirza AF, Mo J, Holt JL, et al. Is There a Relationship between Throbbing Pain and Arterial Pulsations? *J Neurosci*. 2012. doi:10.1523/jneurosci.0193-12.2012

12 LET'S GO WITH BIOLOGY.

Throbbing pain is not throbbing; the brain hurts; the arteries are not swollen or dilated; the Neuroimmune System learns to make mistakes; the brain is indoctrinated... Everything is upside down.

LET'S REFLECT ON basic Biology matters. They will help you understand the nonsense of migraine barbarism. First, you must clearly differentiate the term "pain" from the term "damage". Do you appreciate the difference?

PAIN DOESN'T EQUAL DAMAGE

DAMAGE REFERS TO an objective fact, the loss of the physical integrity of a tissue. On the subject of pain, we will always refer to **necrotic damage**, the violent death of healthy and competent cells.

Biologically (evolutionarily) the Neuroimmune System appears to detect incidences of violent cell death (necrosis) consummated or imminent (there are dangerous agents or states that must be avoided quickly).

If pain appears and there is no consummated or imminent necrosis, we can conclude that the painful feeling is not justified (**unnecessary alertness-protection, erroneous**). If the siren sounds and nothing violent has happened, it is a false alarm, even if the sound is real. One thing is the violent event (theft, collapse, fire) and another the sound of the siren.

Pain (the sound of the siren) is a content of consciousness, private, subjective. You can't see it. It's not objectifiable. It doesn't happen in the area you are feeling it. There may be consummated damage (necrosis) or danger (biological agents or lethal physicochemical states).

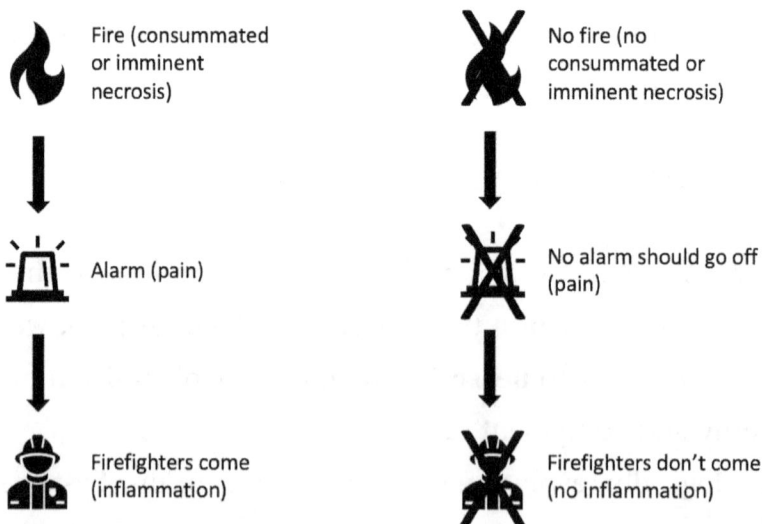

Fire (consummated or imminent necrosis)

Alarm (pain)

Firefighters come (inflammation)

No fire (no consummated or imminent necrosis)

No alarm should go off (pain)

Firefighters don't come (no inflammation)

Let's focus on "necrosis." Don't be afraid of new words.

NECROSIS AND APOPTOSIS

THE ORGANISM IS a society composed of cells and extracellular space. Cellular individuals are born and then die. They get replaced. The cell itself can detect signs of deterioration and activate a program of "suicide", of immolation, to die in a controlled way without causing danger to neighboring cells.

The Neuroimmune System can also detect molecules present in the membrane, which report this decline and activate, from outside, another pathway that leads to death. It wouldn't be suicide but euthanasia.

There are many programs of controlled death, decided by the organism. The best known is *apoptosis*. Yes, another strange word. In Greek it means "fall of the leaf". In autumn the tree decides to get rid of the leaves and activates the *apoptosis*[23] program. The tree doesn't suffer. It protects itself.

Necrosis is a violent death, not decided by the organism or by the cell itself. Death is caused by a biological agent

---

[23] Childs BG, Baker DJ, Kirkland JL, Campisi J, van Deursen JM. Senescence and apoptosis: dueling or complementary cell fates? *EMBO Rep.* 2014. doi:10.15252/embr.201439245

or a harmful physicochemical state. The cell was healthy, competent, with no indicators of decline.

For there to be violent cell death, *necrosis*, there must be **lethal energy**, which can be mechanical (compression, tearing, distension), thermal (burning, freezing) or chemical (acids, lack of blood supply, germs).

If necrosis is consummated, the cell membrane is fragmented, and the contents come out. There's a dangerous chemical release that threatens the lives of healthy neighboring cells. The vigilant cells of the Neuroimmune System detect those internal molecules that have gone outside, and respond quickly, activating *inflammation*, a complex defensive process that minimizes the damage and initiates the regeneration of the destroyed area[24].

---

[24] Roh JS, Sohn DH. Damage-Associated Molecular Patterns in Inflammatory Diseases. *Immune Netw*. 2018. doi:10.4110/in.2018.18.e27

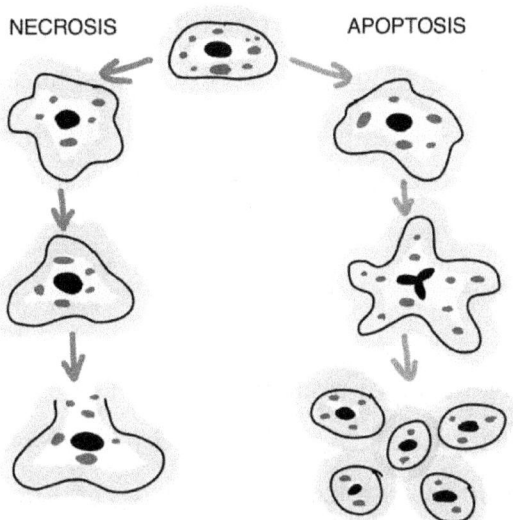

NECROSIS   APOPTOSIS

NOCICEPTORS

THE VIGILANT NEURONS, present in all tissues, the so-called "*nociceptors*" (nocivity receptors)[25], detect the signs of necrosis and encode them in a train of electrical potentials that travel to various neuronal centers, which collaborate in the protection and repair of damaged tissues.

The last layer of processing is the brain. The signals reach a reception area (*primary nociceptive cortex*) and from there are distributed to the "Pain Neuromatrix",

---

[25] Woolf CJ, Ma Q. Nociceptors-Noxious Stimulus Detectors. *Neuron*. 2007. doi:10.1016/j.neuron.2007.07.016

responsible for creating in consciousness the feeling of pain, projected on the area from which the signals arose.

Tissues don't hurt. They get damaged. The Neuroimmune System detects the damage and responds. Pain is the projection to consciousness of that response of the organism, the Neuroimmune System.

Should it only hurt if there's necrosis or danger of necrosis?

With the example of a security system one can answer oneself: Should the alarm only sound if there is an event that justifies the existence of the system: theft, fire, collapse...? That would be ideal. No false positives or negatives.

The function of the Neuroimmune System is not limited to detecting consummated incidents of necrosis. The ideal is to detect the states and agents that can provoke them and neutralize them, before they exert their lethal action.

For this purpose, the Neuroimmune System's vigilant cells are equipped with dangerous state and agent sensors. They inform the evaluation network of their presence and pain may appear without damage having been consummated. Protective responses that neutralize those agents and states are activated and the pain is gone. You can detect the presence of a thief and stop him before he consummates the theft.

I can burn my hand. **Consummated necrosis**. The vigilant cells of the Neuroimmune System detect intracellular molecule leaks. They inform and organize the inflammatory response, foreseeably with the pain projected on consciousness.

I can have my hand over a hot casserole. Thermal danger sensors detect high temperature and inform the response centers. Probably by the time you've felt the pain, those centers have quickly moved your hand away from the casserole. The pain will have been brief. **Imminent damage, not consummated.**

Pain, from the point of view of biological, evolutionary good judgement, should appear in consciousness only when there are incidences of consummated or imminent necrosis. If this is not the case, we would be faced with a threat assessment error, a false positive.

In migraine and other similar labels there is neither consummated nor imminent necrosis. We are dealing with an **autoneuroimmune disease**[26], a threat assessment error, an unnecessary meningeal alert (improperly called "meningitis"). There's actually no inflammation.

---

[26] C L, K Y, A B, D K. Migraine-like headache in bacterial meningitis. *Cephalalgia*. 2000. doi:10.1111/j.1468-2982.2000.00110.x

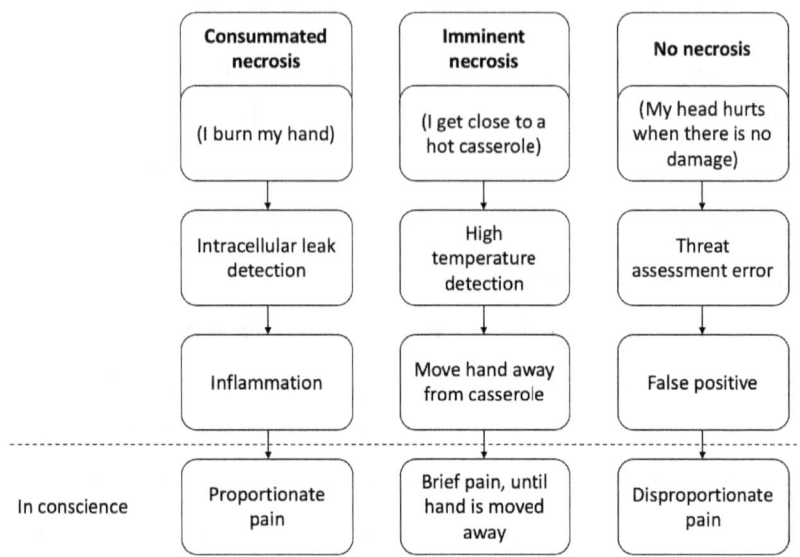

13 THE PAIN PARADIGM SHIFT

The emergence of Neuroscience has substantially changed the theoretical framework from which the professional should evaluate the problem of pain and act accordingly. Not always that necessary change occurs immediately.

DAMAGE IS A matter of tissue. **The tissue is the issue.**

Pain is an evaluative brain issue. **No brain, no pain.**

Already from the middle of the last century, it was obvious, following the confirmation in the Second World War of the lack of correlation between the wounds of the soldiers and the pain they described, that there were other important factors that could, in the face of the same damage, generate more or less pain.

Pain, it began to be suggested, is a complex perception that contains, in variable proportion, tissue stimuli, but also memories, culture, states of attention, predictions, imagination, context, motivation... etc.[27]

Neuroimaging tests have described a wide network of brain areas (the Pain Neuromatrix) whose joint activation is necessary and sufficient for the feeling of pain to appear in the consciousness of an individual, and relates it as the only witness.

Without brain, without consciousness, there is no pain, no other perception. There are no images, no sounds, no smells, no tastes.

Tissue information is constantly reaching the corresponding processing areas. Information from the retina to the "visual neuromatrix"; from the ears to the "auditory neuromatrix"; from neurons sensitive to consummated or imminent damage (nociceptors) to the "pain neuromatrix".

Neuromatrixes do not need the corresponding event information to be activated. They anticipate possible states, predict what may happen, based on previous learning experience. Information from the senses confirms or belies what each neuromatrix anticipates. If there is a non-foreseen novelty, they evaluate the novelty, activate

---

[27] Moseley GL, Butler DS. Fifteen Years of Explaining Pain: The Past, Present, and Future. *J Pain*. 2015. doi:10.1016/j.jpain.2015.05.005

evaluation resources, and fix or divert attention to the novelty.

We can activate each of the neuromatrixes with imagination. I can imagine a face of a specific person and I will activate the same neuromatrix that is activated when I see that face, in a photograph or in physical presence. The only difference is the intensity and persistence of the activation.

The imagined generates a tenuous, fleeting activity. Only when the imagined has more convincing force or relevance for the brain, can it appear with the appearance of reality in the consciousness. Neurophysiologists call it **hallucination: perception without stimulus.** We see a face, but if we take a picture in the space in which we see it, there is no trace of that face. We feel pain, but where it hurts there is no harm to explain and justify it.

CAN ONE IMAGINE THAT IT HURTS AND STARTS HURTING, OR IMAGINE THAT IT DOESN'T HURT AND STOPS HURTING?

THE CONSCIOUS INDIVIDUAL has a limited role in the imaginative process. It needs the collaboration, the approval, the complicity of the unconscious areas, in order to generate a perception with a real appearance.

The placebo effect and the nocebo effect can make the pain go away or appear because of the expectation generated by the information. The neuromatrix can be activated and deactivated with words... as long as we have the approval of the unconscious brain. It is necessary to gain the passage to consciousness and this can only be achieved by having success in the neural social network.

Physiological activation of the neuromatrix occurs when necrosis is consummated or imminent. The signals of damage reach the reception area (primary nociceptive cortex) and from there, immediately, are distributed to all processing areas, which will generate or not, depending on the context, pain in consciousness[28] [29]. In some very empathic individuals, the observation of damage in others is enough to facilitate the perception of pain when applying stimuli[30].

On the contrary, there may be no pain if the damage occurs in a context of real danger, which requires the absence of pain in order to survive. For example, running to escape a fire.

---

[28] Garcia-Larrea L. The posterior insular-opercular region and the search of a primary cortex for pain. *Neurophysiol Clin*. 2012. doi:10.1016/j.neucli.2012.06.001

[29] Garcia-Larrea L, Peyron R. Pain matrices and neuropathic pain matrices: A review. In: *Pain*. ; 2013. doi:10.1016/j.pain.2013.09.001

[30] Godinho F, Faillenot I, Perchet C, Frot M, Magnin M, Garcia-Larrea L. How the pain of others enhances our pain: Searching the cerebral correlates of 'compassional hyperalgesia.' *Eur J Pain*. 2011. doi:10.1002/j.1532-2149.2011.00039.x

In migraines, the erroneous evaluation of imminent damage activates the neuromatrix enough for pain to appear in consciousness, with the same appearance of reality as if something were actually happening (necrosis).

14 TRIGGERS

The "generator" would be a group of genetically hyperexcitable neurons. An evaluative damage neuromatrix, genetically hyperexcitable, indifferent to information, to accumulated experience, with no possibility of change? Um, it doesn't seem very human...
Once the "generator" has been activated, the prolonged hell of the crisis is set in motion, constituting a loop that is difficult to contain.
The triggers (stress, restless sleep, hunger, weekends, weather and hormonal changes, etc.) would turn on the "generator".
That's the official proposal. The possible contribution of the continuous evaluative process, the history that each organism builds on itself, by the warmth of the expert culture, the infosphere of pain, is not contemplated.
Could not that omnipresent story, always available, which consumes most of the energy, be the "generator"?

———————————

A STUDY WAS published in *Neurology*, the official journal of the American Academy of Neurology, in which they tried to provoke a migraine crisis on patients who had identified their triggers, precisely by exposing them to them. It was a failure. They only managed to do so in a meagre 10% of cases[31].

The study resulted in an editorial comment, signed by two of the most renowned experts, suggesting that experimental replication of migraines with triggers can be more complex than it seems. The response to a trigger depends on the **expectation of the response, prior conditions, learning, memory, motivation, and meaning.**

HABITUATION

IF MIGRAINES ARE a brain disorder of habituation to normal sensory signals, shouldn't you rather try to **habituate your brain rather than avoid the trigger?**[32]

The "migrainous" brain is sensitive to absolutely harmless stimuli, agents, states and scenarios. The strategy of identifying and avoiding triggers, as suggested by the authors, could facilitate the anomalous state of awareness and, perhaps, it would be more reasonable to work on habituation to what doesn't contain any danger[33]. When I read the paper and the editorial comment, I thought

---

31 Hougaard A, Amin F, Hauge AW, Ashina M, Olesen J. Provocation of migraine with aura using natural trigger factors. *Neurology*. 2013. doi:10.1212/WNL.0b013e31827f0f10

32 Goadsby PJ, Silberstein SD. Migraine triggers: Harnessing the messages of clinical practice. *Neurology*. 2013. doi:10.1212/WNL.0b013e31827f100c

33 Martin PR. Managing headache triggers: Think "coping" not "avoidance." Cephalalgia. 2010. doi:10.1111/j.1468-2982.2009.01989.x

that something might start to change in the usual coping with migraines, but it didn't.

In another study, its authors advised gradual exposure to triggers and achieved a 50% reduction in days of pain[34]. Expectations, learning, what they have taught the organism, play an important role. Dedicating oneself to identifying the supposed trigger and then avoiding it is not a good proposal.

If, in fact, we have identified a trigger, what we must do is work and dissolve the evaluation that makes it a threat, that is, expose ourselves to it from the conviction that there is no threat.

34 Martin PR, Reece J, Callan M, et al. Behavioral management of the triggers of recurrent headache: A randomized controlled trial. Behav Res Ther. 2014. doi:10.1016/j.brat.2014.07.002

15 THE BRAIN IMAGINES REALITY

The brain imagines, predicts reality. It constantly guesses and contrasts with the information collected by sensory neurons on what is happening inside and outside.
What we perceive is a hallucination controlled by the senses, say neuroscientists.
Nothing happens during a migraine, but the brain acts as if something is happening. It ignores sensory information and lets itself be carried away by its imagination. It is an uncontrolled hallucination, alien to what really happens, that is, nothing.
The "generator" imposes the trigeminal sensitization with its paroxysmal activation and the pain is served, say the neurologists.
The evaluative state imposes the state of alertness-protection with its beliefs and expectations, I propose...

THE ORGANISM IMAGINES itself through the continuous evaluative process and, in that dream, weighs the consequences of the individual's behavior, of its plans in each scenario.

Probably, the most important biological function of the organism is that of constructing a narrative, a history that integrates all the memory of the organism's interaction with the environment and provides a preview of the future, pending validation or modification, with the facts[35].

It is hard to understand why, if nothing is happening, this nonsensical evaluation isn't thwarted. One may be dreaming, but, upon awakening, the contents of the nightmare dissolve. Just open your eyes. One can accept that sleep is a hallucination not controlled by the senses, but it is hard to believe that the brain has nightmares, hallucinations, with open eyes.

The outside world is one thing. We learn to imagine it quite reasonably, with the information provided by the cameras of the eye throughout the learning and the interaction with everything we see, touch, hear, smell and taste.

The dream of our early years gives way to the real world. They can tell us many stories of goblins, giants, monsters, gnomes and unicorns and we will give them credit, but as we mature, we will only believe in what the senses corroborate.

---

[35] Abraham A. The imaginative mind. *Hum Brain Mapp*. 2016. doi:10.1002/hbm.23300

However, the senses can detect stimuli of which stories of uncertain veracity are told. We'll no longer believe in the fantasy stories of childhood, but we can believe in the negative impact of electromagnetic fields, food, environmental toxins, stress, weather changes... In that case, the organism will monitor, detect and respond to what it believes may be threatening. What we see, hear, smell or feel may be assessed as threatening to some, and harmless to others.

The inside of the organism is a different thing. We have sensors that detect dangerous states and agents, but we cannot ensure that our interaction with the outside is not causing negative internal effects, undetectable by those sensors.

The organism will act through the Neuroimmune System from its uncertainties and fears, from the history it has been building, from certain expectations and beliefs. False positives may appear for the first time. The first crisis.

It is fundamental that we think it over, knowing that we are looking at an opaque world, the interior of the organism. There are only cells and extracellular space. Each cell is a complex web of chemical reactions. The activity of the kidneys, lungs, heart, skin, digestive or circulatory system is absolutely unconscious.

We do not know how these processes are taking place, whether digestion is slow or fast, whether arteries are contracted or dilated, what lymphocytes do or the hustle and bustle of the bone marrow. Only when something relevant occurs or, and this is the important thing, when the Neuroimmune System evaluates that it can occur, will we feel this evaluation of the opaque interior, in the form of symptoms.

We feel the pain, the nausea, the sensory intolerance and we talk about the possible causes, using the stories that the experts have previously told us about our insides.

A striking feature of crises is their progression. First, they are pre-felt, and then they begin in the form of increasing pain, vomiting and sensory intolerance. There seems to be nothing that can stop the crisis once it has begun, without resorting to painkillers.

The conscious brain-individual dialogue determines whether the crisis gains strength, is positively fed back or is disrupted. The exit to conscience of the evaluative state expresses the integration of all the processes involved in that evaluation. It only happens when the threat consideration exceeds a threshold of relevance.

The exit to consciousness informs all layers of processing, re-enters and forms a loop. The sound of the siren is picked up by the alarm system. That makes the hypothesis that something threatening is happening stronger. Alert and protection resources are automatically activated. The police come with their sirens to investigate.

There is still one more layer of processing: the consultation of experts. The information they provide is also incorporated into the evaluation process. Loops of all kinds are formed and, if nothing is done, the intensity of activation of the evaluation network increases until it becomes unbearable.

Imagine that the neural network is like a social network. An opinion is continually being generated on each event, regardless of whether or not what is said is true. When something is said to be successful, "the social network is on fire", the flow of information between all the components increases. That would be the access to conscience, the success of a proposal circulating on the net.

The experts are continually dumping information. Individuals, consciously or unconsciously, incorporate that information and the network processes it until one day, it reaches the level of success required and appears in consciousness, expressed as pain: "they said that the head can be destroyed...".

16 PROPORTIONATE AND DISPROPORTIONATE PAIN

How can such intense pain occur if there is nothing abnormal? That's exactly why.

———————————

THERE ARE MODERATE, reasonable pains. They happen in a limited time and place. Proportionate pain accompanies violent tissue destruction events (thermal, mechanical, chemical, infectious). It appears in consciousness hand in hand with the event. It notifies about it. It's forcing us to look into the cause. Once established and controlled, it subsides and remains in the damaged area in the background, protecting it while it is being repaired. Proportionate pain expresses its evolutionary sense, its *raison d'être*.

Disproportionate pain has no containment in space, time or intensity. There's no limit. There is no such thing because, in reality, there is no physical support for the concrete destructive event. If we dig into the area that hurts, we won't find anything.

A migraine crisis is a disproportionate event, unlimited in its mortification. It is announced with an uneasiness that augurs the worst, already known: *crescendo* pain, nausea and sensory intolerance, hopelessness for the fulfillment of the feared, the uncertain and partial relief of therapies, the not knowing what is going on ... or worse: the sentencing of the "migraine" label, an innate irreversible condition, responsible for the storm.

Any hypothesis about its origin must contemplate and explain this excessive dynamic of a process that feeds itself in a spiral, until reaching the maximum level of expression. In the crisis there is a loop, a circular process in which the output is an input that reinforces the next output, something similar to the coupling of an amplification system that initiates a growing beep, which only disappears by lowering the volume of the amplifier or moving the microphone away.

In the official hypothesis, an origin is proposed in the "migraine generator", a supposed set of neurons of hyperexcitable (genetic) condition, which enter into activity causing the trigeminal perivascular terminals to become sensitive and begin to generate "pain signals", as if something were happening. These signals reach the central amplifiers and give an increasing impulse of awareness to the trigeminal terminals. The loop is formed. The painkillers would block the trigeminal sensitizing messengers.

My proposal places the "generator" germ in the fluctuating, learned evaluative states. Each time, place and circumstance gives rise to a state of connectivity that contains an implicit threat assessment. This evaluative state is expressed in consciousness when it reaches a certain level of prediction-fear. At that moment, the conscious individual enters the loop and feeds back, from fear to suffering, the vicious circle. The evaluative state is reinforced in a spiral. The organism exposes in conscience all its arsenal of alertness-protection, in an excessive way, without contention from a harmful reality that sets a limit.

The sensitizers released by the trigeminal are the consequence of the evaluative state. What should be done is dissolve that state, reverse the direction of the spiral. Impose the conviction that nothing is happening. Do we have the power to reverse the vicious spiral? Absolutely not. There is no possibility of ending the process, at will.

However, we can give our conscious contribution. We can provide the information that nothing is happening, focus on our tasks and wish ourselves luck. The students who manage to dissolve the crisis do so. A reader of my book "Migraine, a brain nightmare" tells it like that in a tweet:

"I'm gonna end up going crazy. I'm still halfway through the book, but when the migraine comes, I start talking to myself... and it seems to be going well!"

We all talk to ourselves, but we don't all tell ourselves the same things. In the official proposal, a dialogue with oneself reverberates what has been learned from the instructors and each one's experience. In the proposal of the evaluative error, the dialogue incorporates the discrepant voice of the newly instructed student, who now has the quite probable possibility of reversing the spiral.

Talking to oneself is a continuous, inevitable process. Those who think they don't talk to themselves and just take the painkiller are wrong. They're as crazy as the ones who confess it. This dialogue integrates cognitions, emotions, perceptions and decisions, everything that is contained in the crisis. We have to put measure to what is excessive. Reality:

There's nothing going on. False alarm.

That's all there is to it. It's as simple as that. So uncertain and seemingly inaccessible.

17 In Good Conscience

On the opaque interior, we only have the information projected to consciousness in the form of symptoms and the set of knowledge acquired over that interior, facilitated by the expert culture.
The limited scope for conscious intervention must be optimized. That includes getting rid of the beliefs and expectations of the expert culture, which do not conform to reality.

THE FUNDAMENTAL PROBLEM of understanding pain lies in consciousness. As individuals, we receive on the private dashboard of the organism, on the screen of consciousness, the flow of the continuous evaluative process. It is expressed in the form of thoughts, emotions, perceptions and actions, from a common coding.

We have no idea how the joint activity of the neural network gives rise to those contents of the screen, how the different perceptive qualities (*qualias*) appear: "green", "sweet", a house, a smiling person, pain, sadness. The same goes for ideas and actions.

A neuron is a cell like any other. Its DNA is the same as that of a liver cell. However, the architecture of neural connections gives rise to contents of consciousness and the architecture of hepatic cells gives rise to bile.

Only neural tissues organized as a highly integrated network can generate consciousness. At least that's what it looks like. Only the neural network can make use of the basic memory to share it in that highly integrated network and extract probabilities, generate predictions, imagine, fear, wait, believe, doubt...[36]

All cells memorize, and this allows them to respond differently to the same stimulus. What distinguishes neurons is the socialization of that memory, sharing it on the net. This allows another level of processing.

Muscles don't hurt. They limit themselves to putting up with situations of stress or death and releasing molecular signals that they have suffered damage or are about to suffer damage. The molecular signals of these muscular incidences of danger are captured by the vigilant neurons of the territory and these signals, when entering the socialized network, contribute to generating the content of consciousness that we call pain.

---

[36] Marchetti G. Consciousness: a unique way of processing information. *Cogn Process*. 2018. doi:10.1007/s10339-018-0855-8

Sometimes they send the facts of the tissues, and the signals of damage are enough to ignite the whole defensive net, bringing out in consciousness the feeling of pain. Other times, they send fears, beliefs and expectations. Those fears are also enough to bring out in the same space of consciousness the feeling of pain, after having activated much of the same network that generated the pain by hitting a finger with a hammer.

Professionals should, in good conscience, take conscience into account and spread what we know about it, even if it's not much. Above all, they should explain, in good conscience, that pain always comes from the continuous processing of that socialized memory, constructed by the experience of the individual himself and the observation of the experiences of others, but, above all, by the instruction of experts.

The contents of that instruction do not always correlate with what actually happens in the fabrics, but have more to do with what that *superbrain* of culture imagines, fears, desires, needs, believes, hopes...

We're a social species. Neurons have been organized into a complex network of socialized individual memory. Individuals are organized in a complex network of socialized brains. Pain, in the absence of tissue damage, informs of the contents that this socialized culture introduces into the network of each person. Preventing the risks of such dependence is urgent.

We must appeal to conscience as a neuronal issue that explains the plot of pain and as an ethical issue: the right of citizens to know its importance and, thus, protect themselves from the suffering and disability that that culture, unnecessarily, brings. That culture that ignores or disregards the issue of conscience and bores us with news of genes, serotonins, new drugs ...

In good conscience, let's talk about conscience.

18 NOCICEPTIVE LEARNING

The Neuroimmune System makes mistakes. Each migraine crisis is an undetected and uncorrected error.
Experts say it's a genetic error and overlook learning, schooling.
One is simply born with the so-called "generator", an unstable group of neurons that fire easily and end up sensitizing the trigeminal, giving rise to signals of damage, without there being any.
In my opinion, if something characterizes the neural network is learning, its ability to respond to the conditions of the environment, but one thing is the physical environment and another is the cultural, which enhances an idea of organism against which it is not possible to adapt, but submit to it.

WE ARE THE species that comes into the world with the least competition to survive by our means. We need attention and care over a long period of time.

We are also the only species with organism experts. They inform us of the Anatomy, Physiology and Pathology of our Apparatus and Systems, of what is convenient and inconvenient. They interpret our symptoms, organize syndromes, diagnostic labels, and prescribe remedies. We can't do anything but trust what they tell us. We can't figure out for ourselves how the body works.

THE FIRST CRISIS

ONE BAD DAY, the first headache crisis appears. We ask the doctor, and from that moment on, we're in her hands. Patients go through traditional and alternative medicine consultations and believe in what relieves their pain or what they *wish* was true (*wishful thinking*). The shocking thing about this pilgrimage is that, probably, nobody has told you about what we are talking about here, about the errors in the evaluation of the Neuroimmune System. Nor will they have considered the possibility that those mistakes can be learned. There's only room for pathology. Something must be sick and must be corrected.

LEARNING

THERE REALLY IS no Biology without learning. All living things learn. They act, memorize what they have done, the positive and negative consequences of their actions, and repeat or modify their behavior depending on how it went. We learn from our own experience, from injuries, infections, burns, intoxications... Just as we need eyes to learn to see, we need *nociceptors* (neurons that detect consummated or imminent damage) to dynamize defensive learning.

EXPERIENCE

ONE'S OWN EXPERIENCE of damage can lead to awareness, fear of further damage, hypervigilance, avoidance... or the opposite: hardening, habituation to moderate damage, as it happens in sports. The stress tolerance band, the risk, is plastic.

In addition to our own experience, we can shape our style of alertness-protection, observing the damage of others, imitating models in our parents. We are a very imitative species, with a prolonged dependence on the caregiver model. Not only do we receive genes from parents, which push us towards an explorer mode with risk acceptance or the opposite: avoidance of harm, fearful or vigilant behavior... but we observe and imitate what we see in our predecessors [37] .

---

[37] Noel M, Beals-Erickson SE, Law EF, Alberts NM, Palermo TM. Characterizing the pain narratives of parents of youth with chronic pain. *Clin J Pain*. 2016. doi:10.1097/AJP.0000000000000346

MIGRAINE ISN'T TRANSMITTED. IT'S RETRANSMITTED.

IT IS POSSIBLE that those genes that push us to the avoidant mode, with the upbringing in a family in which some member suffers crises, get strengthened. In that family, the learned interpretation that the first crisis of a descendant confirms that he has received the genes of the disease, will prevail. And that he is condemned to suffer what he has already seen in a parent.

It is fundamental, in these cases, to reduce the weight of genetics and to present the fundamental role of breeding in an environment that promotes, without being aware of it, the unnecessary states of alertness-protection that characterize the label "migraine". "He has inherited it from his mother" can and should be replaced by "he has learned it from his mother", who, in turn, has learned it from the expert culture that exclusively limits the role of family transmission to what genes determine and overlooks the educational factor, with imitation as a fundamental element.

Experts

Finally, in our species, we have experts dedicated to studying biological processes, with greater or lesser fortune. Maybe what's being told about migraines is, at least, questionable.

There is much new knowledge available on the role of the defensive neural network, on the imaginative-predictive brain, the importance of beliefs and expectations, the impact of culture on nociceptive learning. Ignoring the educational factor, instructor-led parenting, is doing patients a disservice.

The official culture of the "migraine" label is sensitizing, promotes vigilance, alertness, avoidance, dependence on therapies, conviction of pathology, mystery, hopelessness, fear. One possible proof of this is the high incidence of migraines in neurologists (those who propose the official expert culture)[38] [39]. Primary care physicians, however, have an incidence similar to that of non-professionals[40] .

---

[38] Evans RW, Lipton RB, Silberstein SD. The prevalence of migraine in neurologists. *Neurology*. 2003.
doi:10.1212/01.WNL.0000090628.46508.D4

[39] Alstadhaug KB, Hernandez A, Næss H, Stovner LJ. Migraine among Norwegian neurologists. *Headache*. 2012. doi:10.1111/j.1526-4610.2012.02216.x

[40] Waters WE. Migraine in general practitioners. *Br J Prev Soc Med*. 1975. doi:10.1136/jech.29.1.48

The narrative that every organism builds on itself is marked by what the experts say about that organism.

In our migraine courses, we expose this proposal of the evaluative error, supported in what science is finding out about the Neurophysiology of brain activity. The brain misprocesses information, they say. In my opinion, the brain, the neural network, does its work guided not by a pathological, genetic, hyperexcitability condition but by a sensitizing information that imposes the state of alertness-protection and does not allow its correction.

The brain processes well... the available information.

19 SELF-FULFILLING PROPHECY

Migraine starts many times in childhood. It can be expressed as a crisis of abdominal pain, of a limb, as recurrent episodes of vertigo or as spasmodic torticollis, before modeling itself as the typical adult migraine.

The migraine sufferer parent will think she's passed on her disease genetics. She'll try to protect, watch, sensitize, to minimize the drama. She may even have a bad conscience for having brought into the world a child condemned to migraine mortification.

THE APPEARANCE OF crises in the offspring of a parent stigmatized by migraine confirms the worst predictions: she has transmitted the sick condition to her son and has therefore condemned him to a life cut short by crises. The expert consultation only corroborates what is already feared, but there is always the possibility of something new in the advice and therapies.

"It is indeed a migraine. You passed on your genes to your son. You should educate him in healthy, orderly lifestyles, in the early use of painkillers. In the immediate future, we may finally have new, more precise and specific treatments. We'll keep you posted."

It seems that the approach has not changed: the same prophecy, the reference to new treatments. What was feared seems to have been fulfilled. Crises come hand in hand with genes, of hyperexcitable generators. The problem may be acceptably controlled, but it may also initiate uncontrollable dynamics. Everything reinforces the belief that migraine is a genetic issue against which little or nothing can be done.

From the proposal of the learned evaluative error, the question is seen in a different, opposite way. Genes act in a complex way. Each gene influences several factors and each factor is influenced by several genes. There is no such thing as a migraine gene, except in very rare family forms. The genome has a long way to go before it ends up expressing itself in one way or another.

The environment, the breeding, the habitat influence powerfully. In matters of the brain, we must not lose sight of the learning, the contents of the expert culture, the idea of organism that each organism makes itself, depending on how it comes into the world and runs through it.

Remember: the zip code is more important, in this case and in many others, than the genetic code.

From the learned model we would explain:

We do not know exactly what genetics you have transmitted to your child, what conditions it generates and how it will express itself. You could have transmitted to him, for example, a tendency to obey, to promote strategies of avoidance of harm, to gregarious conduct...

What you won't be able to avoid is the genetics of learning, in a species like ours, which requires a long period of dependence on caregivers who will mark the paths along which to circulate. In this matter, the path is made before you, but one very well signposted and fenced, without alternatives. It is the one that leads to the maturity of the migraine, to the state of unjustified alertness-protection, to false positives.

"There is no way of knowing what you have genetically transmitted to your child. It is easier to detect what has been transmitted to him, simply, unconsciously, by observation-imitation, as a model of what could happen to him in the future, as an educational guideline of overprotection, covert alarmism, drug dependence, medicalization, in short."

"Your child will reside in a healthy organism, but will be protected by an alarmist, sensitized, hypervigilant, fearful, mistaken, irrational Neuroimmune System. Believing to the hilt in what it has been indoctrinated, or on the contrary: a sensible, permissive Neuroimmune System, enlightened in its own dangers, aware of the risks of expert culture and of the importance of learning."

Prophecy can be thwarted as soon as one discovers the importance of instructor-led learning. Migraine sufferer parents who attend courses with their children understand the danger, turn their role as care-instructors 180 degrees and manage, in many cases, to rid their offspring of the nonsense of migraines.

20 REWARD SYSTEM

The organism weaves and unweaves its history, through its own experience, the observation of others and the instruction of experts, and expresses itself on the screen of consciousness in the form of symptoms.
Consciousness reflects the evaluative state of each scenario, but also the intentionality burden of the organism.
The individual must collaborate by accepting a behavior consistent with what the Neuroimmune System requests.
But for that, it has to be willing to do it. This is also done by the Neuroimmune System itself.

THE SKIN IS an organ potentially threatened by parasites or toxic chemicals. The Neuroimmune System ensures its integrity with sensors capable of detecting various types of threats. If it detects stimuli assessed as "dangerous," it needs the individual to **want to** scratch herself to remove it from the skin. It could be a parasite or a toxic molecule.

The itching fulfills this function: it expresses in conscience the urgent proposal that the individual gets a

desire to scratch. All the symptoms contain this double facet: the evaluative and the behavioral proposal. Each symptom contains the urge towards a certain behavior: hunger proposes to eat; thirst, to drink; tiredness, to rest; itching, to scratch; nausea, to vomit; sensory intolerance, to stay in the den.

The so-called Motivational System or Punishment-Reward System is in charge of setting certain desires that force the individual to do what the evaluative state of each scenario establishes[41].

Dopamine is the messenger that orders the neural network to activate the desire for this or that. If a behavior is evaluated as convenient by the evaluative network, dopamine will be released to memorize and enhance that behavior. That way, it will be repeated if we expose ourselves to the same scenario. Behaviors that follow a negative impact will be memorized by removing the *dopamine* seal and they will be avoided.

The Motivational System is faithful to what the evaluation network dictates. If culture imposes the habit of smoking, there is no point in dying with the first cigarettes of a teenager. The cultural mandate requires overcoming these drawbacks. Dopamine will seal the

---

[41] Porreca F, Navratilova E. Reward, motivation, and emotion of pain and its relief. *Pain*. 2017. doi:10.1097/j.pain.0000000000000798

engagement and the novice, in the toxic habit of tobacco, will not be able to avoid the desire, the temptation to light another cigarette. If the behavior required by the Motivational System is not executed, the pressure increases, and the individual may end up bowing to the **desire.**

The action of taking a sedative in a crisis is demanded by the Motivational System, based on an evaluative state of threat that impels the desire to take the pill[42].

Rebellion can succeed if it is based on a strong conviction that the threat assessment is absurd. The individual does not listen to the proposal of his organism and does not fulfill its desires... **because he does not feel like it.** It can work, but not always.

---

[42] Auvray M, Myin E, Spence C. The sensory-discriminative and affective-motivational aspects of pain. *Neurosci Biobehav Rev.* 2010. doi:10.1016/j.neubiorev.2008.07.008

21 THE WORKSHOP OF CONSCIOUSNESS

The face is the mirror of the soul. Consciousness is the mirror of the organism. It expresses what this ongoing evaluation process is up to.
The individual recognizes, through symptoms, the emotional states of her organism, of her Neuroimmune System.
Pain, nausea and sensory intolerance reveal a state of alertness-protection, centered on the head.

THE CRISES EXPRESS in consciousness the fear of the Neuroimmune System to necrotic damage in the head. We come into the world with fear written on the circuits, in charge of watching and protecting. Fear of snakes, rodents, spiders, closed spaces, open spaces, fear of cliffs, stage fright... are fears with biological meaning. They help us stay alive.

In addition to the external threat, there are internal threats. Pathogenic germs may enter; some of your own cells may become cancerous; the ducts may become blocked. The organism, through the Neuroimmune System, monitors these incidents and activates the alarms when it evaluates, rightly and wrongly, that a threat may occur. The fears of the organism are expressed in the consciousness as symptoms. In migraine: pain, vomiting and sensory intolerance.

The patient is not afraid of harm. Her fear focuses on suffering. She is attentive to the emergence of the crisis and its evolution, to the consequences on its agenda. Her fears are well founded. They're totally logical.

Once the crisis begins, the fear of the patient, her vigilant attitude, feedback the evaluative dynamics, contribute to strengthening the spiral. It would be good if the two fears could be dissolved, that of the organism to harm and that of the individual to suffering. Fears produce sensitization to harmless scenarios. What should be tolerated, accustomed to, is sensitized.

WHAT CAN THE PATIENT DO IN THE FACE OF THESE TWO FEARS?

THE BATTLE IS fought in consciousness. It is the workshop in which the patient can contribute her knowledge, internalize it: nothing is happening, and nothing is going to happen. It's a false alarm. The brain isn't sick. There is no pathological condition of hyperexcitability. Only expectations and beliefs that nurture that neural excitement.

In the realm of consciousness, we can make decisions (painkillers yes or no; I continue with my plans to go to dinner or I don't), focus attention on our tasks and divert them from the organism. It's easy to say, but pain can sometimes impose its law.

We can do what we can do, try to impose rationality, dissolve what is imagined, both on the part of the individual and on the part of the organism, so that reality triumphs: false alarm, in spite of all the noise.

Knowledge is the fundamental weapon. If we could run checks on the inside, it would be easier. But, unfortunately, we cannot observe. We have to imagine it not in a capricious way, at will, but trying to impose, with absolute conviction, the hypothesis that there is no situation that justifies the activated state of alertness-protection.

There's no injured or swollen tissue. Just a few circuits where fear has triggered the alarm.

22 FROM THEORY TO PRACTICE

Migraine is learned. It makes sense. The hypothesis is accepted.
What's next?
What can be done to modify the beliefs of a group of neurons that dance to the sound of their memories and predictions, without caring about the damage they can cause to the individual?
The brain secretes pain, but it doesn't suffer it. Mortification rests with the individual.
They say that the brain defends what it believes with all its might, as if they were going to steal from it what is most precious: its history, its story.
How do we convince an enemy that it's deeply mistaken?
The brain, my brain, is my enemy?

THEY SAY THAT the organism is formed by several armies of cellular idiots who do their work blindly, obeying the messages that reach them through the circulatory network (hormones) and the neuronal network (neurotransmitters). There are no feelings, no bad conscience, not even conscience. I have no idea how the contents of consciousness, in this case those of a migraine crisis, can emerge from this complex universe of chemical processes, organized in complex networks.

The fact is that the connectivity on which the continuous evaluative function is based gives rise to this crisis, based on the existence of beliefs and expectations, memories and predictions, motives, fears and desires. The patient only has the conscious space to try to modify the evaluative errors. In that space, there is no point in pleading, appealing to compassion:

"Brain, please have mercy. Don't hurt me..."

Or self-deception, "not noticing":

"I'm going to think it's not hurting..."

The state of alertness-protection demands the attention and collaboration of the conscious individual towards questions of physical security of the head.

What we have to try is to internalize reality, common sense:

"Come on, brain, nothing that you're afraid of is actually happening or is going to happen. Don't panic again. Let me concentrate on my things."

The aim is to influence the evaluation process. Something like hypnosis. The hypnotist should be the conscious individual and the receiver of suggestions, the brain. But the roles may be reversed. There are patients who avoid the dialogue with the brain and opt for giving it the finger.

"The pain used to wake me up. I had to get up, take ibuprofen, but there was nothing left to do. That day I would have a horrible time. Now I say to myself: come on, I'm sleepy! I turn around and go back to sleep. Now, I wake up without pain."

False alarm; evaluative error; cultural indoctrination; automated connectivity, learned. That's the reality. The evaluative state of threat urges the patient, through the desire projected by the motivational system, to take the painkiller.

"If I don't take it, I'll have a very bad day. If I take it, the pain may go away. It'll do something."

It's not a matter of altered chemistry. Although it is true that the CGRP (Calcitonin Gene-Related Peptide) is high and can contribute to sensitize the trigeminal terminals, this is due to the fact that it operates the state of alertness-protection, which provides protection resources in advance in the "threatened" tissues, anticipating a necrosis incident. The CGRP is a messenger that prepares the tissues in advance to start the repair. It is released by the effect of the evaluative state, in the case of migraine, without any justification.

When faced with an evaluative error, it is appropriate to classify it as an error and ensure that the probability of another similar error is minimal.

Being in the eye of the hurricane of a crisis is no easy task. It is understandable to resort to the painkiller if doing so relieves suffering, but we must know that the molecule of the painkiller has not dissolved the pain, but the compliance with a requirement of the evaluative state.

Sometimes, after a frustrated attempt to fight the brain error without submitting to the demand of the painkiller, the patient can't take it anymore or has to attend an event, and decides to give up. In some cases, the pain magically disappears in a couple of minutes. Other times, the patient holds on. He has a hard time, but the pain just goes away.

"I confirmed that the painkiller is not necessary for the pain to go away."

It's a game, an exploration. Doing different things and observing. Learning opportunities must be created, supported by the conviction that the head is not taking any risk and that, if we keep thinking, fearing and doing the same thing, everything will remain the same... or worse.

23 PLASTICITY

Santiago Ramón y Cajal said that everyone can be the sculptor of their own brain, if they wish.
We are born with a certain connectivity only in part. Throughout the learning process, we must measure very diverse and changing environments and have connective states in the network, which respond adaptively to each scenario.
Much of the connectivity is temporary. It can and must be corrected.
Biology is plastic, it adapts.
It learns.

SOME PATIENTS HAVE been suffering from migraine for many years. They think that neural pathways are too steeped to wait for things to change. It's chronic, they think, and that sounds fatal, irreversible.

That's not true. Each connection point (*synapse*) has to prove every day that it's good for something, that it is part of the winning circuits. If there is no activity at that point, the cells of the microglia (the Immune System installed in the Nervous System) eat the synaptic structure, while in areas with more activity demand, new connection points arise. There's a competition to connect. Every point is contested.

The success of connectivity patterns depends on many factors. Of course, of what is happening, of the activity: the map of the cerebral cortex representing the activity of the fingers of the left hand on a violinist increases with practice and decreases if it is abandoned. The hippocampus, the GPS of the brain, increases in size in London taxi drivers. Just as activity produces increased muscle volume, the density of neural connectivity increases when it has to work.

Not only activity induces plastic changes. Imagination, information, thought, dreams, are accompanied by an updating of connectivity patterns and that property remains until death.

It's never too late to change. If the brain resists change, it is not because plasticity has expired due to old age, but because it is stubborn...

24 RESISTANCE

The neural network is a disputed space of connectivity. Each connection point (synapse) must earn the right to remain active.
In each scenario, a pattern of connections wins, and it's the one that arises to conscience, expressed in symptoms.
Novel proposals can be well received if there is boredom and frustration after trying everything. However, many times, the dominant connectivity patterns not only do not give up their power, but reinforce it when something wants to make it seem an erroneous pattern.

FIRST WE DECIDE and then we look for reasons. Something pushes us to make a decision and, once made, we look for arguments to justify it.

The evaluation process also follows this dynamic. It generates contents of conscience and then searches its archives to see if it finds an argument that reinforces the decision already taken. Objections appear, sometimes in the form of unanswered questions. A classic:

"I didn't know what migraines were until I had the first crisis. Why?"

There's no way of knowing. We can construct more or less plausible hypotheses, but we only know that, that day, what was cooked in the net got the force of becoming a symptom in conscience. Another no less classic:

"The pain wakes me up. I wasn't thinking about it. I was sleeping."

The evaluative flow is continuous. It doesn't stop. It delves into the past and the future, imagining possible events of different probability. Consciousness is turned off and on, depending on the physiological cycles and what happens in real time or it imagines in an uncertain moment. If you are turned off (asleep), you can be turned on (wake up) if evaluative rumination considers threat.

If, at that moment, you return to the world in a state of alertness-protection of the organism, you will receive in consciousness the reflection of that state: pain. It is the same thing: to internalize the false alarm and try to keep on sleeping. That's the theory.

The aim is that no argument is made against the evaluative hypothesis, based on the fact that, if one is asleep, one does not think. Then, what is proposed can't be true, in that case.

"While I'm asleep, I don't think, then it can't hurt because I think..."

We must clearly separate the realm of the unconscious, the opacity of complex biological processes, from the space of the conscious. We must work in this universe from knowledge and the will to act in a novel, exploratory way.

25 IT'S WORKING!

The new theoretical framework: there is no disease but error; what is learned can be unlearned...it generates suspense.
Will it work?
The theory is accepted. At least it has a logic, but what can be done to modify the power of dominant connectivity patterns?

STUDENTS DO WHAT they can. Listen, read, reflect, decide to change strategy. They avoid avoidance, expose themselves, explore, play. Just in case, they carry the painkiller in their bag, but they have decided to face the next crisis by refusing to take it.

We have many migraine courses on our backs and the results are quite constant: between 65 and 70% overall reduction of days of pain in all groups; reduction of a couple of points in the intensity; collapse of the consumption of painkillers; recovery of habits lost through fear and, most importantly, knowing that it is not one who causes this nonsense, but learning guided by instructors.

It is neither necessary nor sufficient to learn the lesson well. There is no exam to see if you have worked well and can access a degree. We provide information, food, and wish you luck in the digestive process.

There are times when the evaluative error is dissolved as if by magic.

"I've never had a crisis again."

In others, the error remains valid, only in specific scenarios.

"I'm doing well, but I can't get rid of the crisis that catches me sleeping."

Triggers lose power:

"I have a couple of wine glasses; I go to dinner: I tolerate noisy environments; the weather changes now seem indifferent to me."

The menstrual cycle sometimes resists, but in many cases the pelvic pain and headache dissolve.

There are those who would get an A on a supposed test, but everything remains the same. Maybe there's an overzealousness, knowing everything, putting too much pressure. Ironically, the more you demand of your neural network, the less you get.

"Don't think of a pink elephant for five minutes..."

It's not easy to get rid of the elephant.

There are those who apparently have not understood anything, but have stopped suffering the crises. Probably the evaluation process has admitted the error, in a simple way, and has ceased to have access to the conscience, because the hypothesis of the threat has lost strength.

Failure does not disqualify the validity of the educational proposal.

The concepts we explain are validated by Neuroscience.

"It doesn't work for me. I knew that you couldn't get rid of this just by talking..."

Conviction may be firm, but error resists and does not bend so easily.

"It took me my time. It was hard, but it was worth it."

Students ask for guidelines, methods. They ask for advice.

"What do you think of mindfulness, yoga...?"

Every organism is a different world. Each story is unique, although the contents of the culture are the same. I don't know a strategy that works for everyone. There remains a path of exploratory play that each of us must follow, depending on our style of confrontation, our imaginative capacity.

We must flee from the feeling of guilt.

"Why does it work for others and not for me? I must be doing something wrong."

Don't mortify yourself. Keep trying, without anguish, without anxiety, without haste...

26 PAINKILLERS

"I tried to talk to my brain, not to be aware of the pain, to internalize the idea that nothing was going on inside my head, that it was a false alarm, but the pain became unbearable and I resorted to the painkiller."

PAINKILLERS AREN'T MAGIC molecules. Much of their effect is due to what is expected of them.

WITH DAMAGE

SUPPOSE I HAVE just sprained my ankle.

"I feel pain in my ankle."

The healthy terminals of the nociceptive neurons in the area have captured the molecular signals of violent death (*necrosis*) and have codified them in a train of electrical potentials, which is led to various processing-response centers, the last of which is the "evaluative neuromatrix," which ends up expressing itself in the consciousness as "pain", projected on your ankle.

We take an ibuprofen and the pain subsides. What happened?

Very simple: the painkiller has sabotaged the ankle event information, preventing the information from reaching the complex network that processes it and that generates the painful feeling. We can get rid of the information in the terminals of the vigilant neurons, with local anaesthetics, or the activation of the final processing network (evaluative neuromatrix) with general anaesthesia. Less drastically, we've reduced the damage signal train with ibuprofen. The brain network will receive tuned news of the event, making the evaluative neuromatrix see that there is less damage than there really is. The result, deceptive: less pain. Logically, the inflammatory response, repairing the damage, will also be less...

What would be the effect of morphine?

In the first damage information relay station, morphine would prevent traffic of damage signals to areas of the evaluative neuromatrix that generate the affective component (suffering) of pain.

In all cases, we have not acted directly on the pain, since it only exists in the mysterious space of consciousness, but on the chemistry of the generation and trafficking of the message of harm. We can hide or manipulate the information so it hurts less.

WITHOUT DAMAGE

NOW LET'S SUPPOSE there's no damage to the ankle, but it hurts... and a lot. Kind of like an ankle migraine.

"It hurts so much. It's been like this for years. Painkillers don't work for me."

"You've got nothing on your ankle. It shouldn't hurt. The painkillers should have taken away the pain. Maybe it's psychological."

Actually the painkillers, the molecules that sabotaged the damage information, are useless when there is none, for the simple reason that there are no signals to sabotage. They have nowhere to act.

"Not even morphine does anything to me."

We now know that pain is not "psychological" in the usual sense of the term. It occurs in the defensive neural network as a result of a complex evaluative process in which memories, expectations, beliefs, fears, desires... are merged. That is: what rules is the virtual organism.

In this case, analgesic-antinflammatory drugs cannot do anything beyond placebo. The same goes for other drugs.

It's a matter of "central sensitization," they say. Neurons process information badly. In order for them to process better, their excitability is inhibited with antiepileptics, antidepressants, anxiolytics... Placebos? It doesn't matter. The thing is that the "analgesic" action works. Anything goes.

No pain, no pain.

I remind you of Ramachandran's statement: "pain is an opinion". Perhaps, you should try to correct the mistake. Evaluation error detection. Pedagogy. Take away the fear of living.

Pain is an effect. You have to go to the cause: no damage. Processing error, due to erroneous beliefs and expectations, plausibly promoted by the alarmist culture, by the culture of painkillers as a primary tool.

"It hurts."

"There's nothing wrong with your ankle. We're going to try to correct the evaluative error. That ankle doesn't need the state of alertness-protection. What it needs is for the brain to promote its unrestricted activity. Come on, let's run!"

In the head, same thing: Come on, let's live!

27 SOMETHING CHANGES

We organize courses for migraine patients, either in four one-and-a-half hour classes per week or in a single intensive eight-hour session.
In the weekly classes, the students intervene to tell their experiences from this new framework.
Some have already noticed changes...

STUDENTS HAVE ALREADY learned that migraine is the consequence of a threat assessment error from the brain, similar to that of allergy. They know that pain is one thing and damage is another. They no longer look for triggers and, if they had them, they try to stand up to them: they drink that forbidden wine.

They are comforted to know that it is not they who provoke the crises, but their organism, their overprotective brain. A story like this is not uncommon:

"The pain started. I thought about what I had learned. "Nothing's going on; it's a false alarm." I concentrated on what I was doing. Before, I would have taken the pain-killer and would have tried to take refuge in a quiet environment, without stimuli. Soon the pain was gone."

This can also happen:

"I tried to concentrate on the fact that there was no damage, no danger, and I didn't take the painkiller, but the pain got worse and I had no choice but to resort to ibuprofen."

In both cases they refer to a dialogue with the brain:

"I spoke to my brain..."

It is important to discover that area of consciousness in which the organism projects its evaluative states, converted into symptoms.

That is the space for intervention, and we have two powerful tools:

1) Knowledge. The conviction that symptoms are the expression of that story built on learning.

2) The will, the possibility of managing attention and deciding on our behavior; taking or not taking painkillers; going to dinner; having a glass of wine without fear...[43]

---

[43] Malfliet A, Kregel J, Coppieters I, et al. Effect of pain neuroscience education combined with cognition-targeted motor control training on chronic spinal pain a randomized clinical trial. *JAMA Neurol*. 2018. doi:10.1001/jamaneurol.2018.0492

Actually, we're always talking to the brain, only we're not aware of it. We believe that what we think and decide belongs to us, that the "I" is something with a life of its own, autonomous. Nothing could be further from the truth. The "I" is only the mirror of the evaluative process, an interactive process that allows and promotes our participation.

Usually, the dialogue with the brain is one of consensus, but there are times when we must correct the history that generates the symptoms, given that the brain is acting from an erroneous, irrational, phobic script. Through inner knowledge, we can try to modify beliefs and expectations. There are no magic words, no paths, no guidelines. Each person finds his or her own way of doing it.

"I know there's nothing going on. I just do my thing."

A patient once told me: "When the pain starts, I call for the common-sense anti-pain brigade."

The brain contains an integrated history of the individual's interaction with the environment. It's not a zombie, locked in a cranial box, who imagines reality with its mind. It is the individual who has nourished day by day that story that boils in the brain circuits. The brain is the historical individual.

That's all there is to it.

28 UPS AND DOWNS

IT LOOKED LIKE it was going well. A whole month without pain, something absolutely exceptional, but... the damned crisis reappeared, even more forcefully than ever. The brain doesn't have a recycling bin, shredder, or garbage can. There's only a storage room and a home to live in.

Consciousness feeds on what has earned the right to occupy the useful square meters, but the storage room is overflowing with cognitive, emotional, behavioral junk.

From time to time, and depending on factors foreseeably unknown, the destiny of the mental junk of the storage room is reconsidered and one returns to past times, which, even when they are painful for the individual, can be more reassuring for the defensive net.

You have to count on that eventuality and not fall apart. The question remains the same, the competition between two conflicting evaluative frameworks: that of the mysterious disease, genetics and lifestyle, as opposed to the sensitizing, intolerant learning. Whatever happens, the basic ideas that I have presented in this book and in the courses are still true. The acquired defensive neural network can make mistakes, as can its Immune equivalent.

Ignoring learning with its share of error and its cultural dependence and reducing the problem to supposed genes, the over-stimulation of modern life and unhealthy habits, is ignoring the powerful factor of expert information. Delegating the resolution of the problem to therapies makes it fester.

From the framework that I propose, the moment of the first crisis is fundamental. The professional will probably apply the label "migraine" with everything that goes with it. He'll give some advice and prescribe some painkillers. Maybe everything will go apparently well, and you won't ask for more. Everything may twist and end up in a well of mortification, hopelessness and disability.

If you've visited this book, you probably didn't do very well with the official and alternative proposals. I hope I was right to explain the ABCs of Neuroimmune Defensive Biology. I can only wish you luck.

You, your genes and your lifestyle have done nothing to deserve this.

29 UNLEARNING

Montse decided, tired of trying all the known therapies, to bet on the path of knowledge. Let's go back to her story.

I REMEMBER THAT the first thing I did was go out in the garden and read in the sun without glasses or a hat to protect me. What did I have to protect myself from? The sun? The truth is, it seemed absurd. So, I began to challenge my brain to see who would win, it or me. I did the same thing with each of my migraine triggers. One by one, I faced them with conviction and without fear. Sometimes I was victorious, sometimes I wasn't. But all those personality traits I had always been told were predisposing me to having a migraine? I used them to get rid of it.

LONG LIVE PERFECTIONISM!

BECAUSE YES, I am "too" perfectionist, responsible, organized and stubborn. But those qualities that both doctors and psychologists insisted on changing, have helped us to live without pain. My daughter and I started reading, studying, challenging our brains and talking to them. Sounds weird, I know. We had to convince them that there was no need to continually assess threats that did not exist. Sunshine, sushi, chocolate, staying up late, some alcohol or napping are not threats, it's just living. And that's what my daughter and I started to do, to live.

We then attended a course taught by Dr. Goicoechea. I had already improved quite a lot. The dizziness had completely disappeared, and the migraines had decreased both in frequency and intensity. But my daughter remained the same, with daily pain and dizziness. The course helped us a lot. Hearing from the voice of a neurologist what exactly migraine is and knowing the mechanisms that provoke it gave us, on the one hand, updated knowledge about the biology of pain and on the other, not less important, hope. In addition, sharing our migraine-related experiences with other patients helped us a great deal. We felt understood and accompanied.

Knowledge and hope have been the two key words in my migraine unlearning process. Knowledge cancels out uncertainty and has helped us replace erroneous beliefs that unjustifiably set off an alarm in our brain with new, non-alarmist and truthful information. Hope has allowed us to change a state of discouragement and frustration for positive emotions that have given us strength and perseverance to fight. Because in this process of unlearning migraine, not everything is joyful. There are ups and downs, as in all areas of life.

After the course, we continued learning and practicing. Words like pain, damage, necrosis, nociceptors, threat assessment, defensive warning programs, reward system, mirror neurons, allodynia or efferent copy became part of our lives. We have read and heard everything: biology, neurology, quantum physics, psychology... everything that has reached our hands related to pain and the brain. The theory is simple, but convincing our brain that there's no damage and that, therefore, it doesn't have to activate defensive alert programs when it's not the right time, hasn't been easy. However, over time, our level of awareness has been corrected and we have gradually regained **a life that was hijacked by migraine.**

You're wondering what exactly needs to be done to achieve this. It's a question I kept asking myself. The theoretical framework proposed by Dr. Goicoechea is perfectly understandable and most patients believe it with conviction right away. But then, how can we correct that evaluative error? I guess every person has to find their own way. In my case, as I have already told you, the first thing I did was to put new knowledge into my brain, which would replace the old ideas about migraine: to read, to underline, to reflect. In short, to learn about the Biology of pain. At the same time, I began to change habits to desensitize myself and lose the fear of having a migraine. I learned not to worry about everything and not to plan so much depending on whether or not I had a migraine. I bravely and courageously faced my fears. Each week, I faced a trigger to get used to it. I never went back to the darkroom. I kept telling myself that I was fine, that there was no danger.

I was visualizing my healthy brain. I noticed the people around me without pain and copied their attitudes, their way of doing things, imagining that I didn't have it either. I took a lot of pictures of myself when I managed to overcome the migraine and so, when I couldn't, I looked at the pictures to remind my brain what sensation and emotional state it should have. I exchanged painful and frustrating memories for new positive experiences. Above all,

I was very optimistic and confident that I could unlearn the migraine. And I made it.

A GOOD TEACHER AND TWO GOOD STUDENTS

THROUGHOUT THESE TWO years, I have transmitted to my daughters the importance of learning. I have provided them with a new environment in which they learn not to avoid that which causes us headaches, not to lock themselves in the dark room, not to take a painkiller at the slightest sign. Just as they copied from my beliefs and customs that led them to suffer from migraine, I hope that from now on they will learn to manage pain in a more reasonable, healthy and efficient way. They don't suffer from migraines anymore either.

Knowing the biology of pain at the beginning of my migraine story would have saved me and my family a lot of suffering. Fear, awareness, hypervigilance or avoidance would have had no place in my life. Understanding the reason for pain would have helped us know how to act to deal with it. We would not have given in to false beliefs or copied attitudes and behaviors that fueled our migraine, and I am convinced that my relationship with migraine would have been much shorter.

ACKNOWLEDGEMENTS

I HEARTILY THANK Dr. Goicoechea, Maite Goicoechea, María Jiménez, and all the professionals who work and research day by day so that the knowledge of pain biology reaches all of us and helps us to prevent unnecessary uncertainty, suffering and pain. I also thank all those I have met on this path of "healing" and with whom I have shared joys and defeats.

30 LEARNING AND COPING

EACH PATIENT MUST explore, from the conviction that nothing threatening happens in the head, the way to disrupt the scary movie that the evaluative neuromatrix is playing. Nothing we feel responds to reality. As a spectator of that film, we interact with its plot and we can modify the script, making it have a happy ending.

These are coping testimonies that were collected from some students:

LEARNING AND REVIEWING

- I read the book or I attended the course once and it worked. I didn't need anything else.

- I have underlined book phrases to review when needed.

- I read and learn the concepts well.

- I watch conferences or talks on YouTube by Arturo Goicoechea.

- I see short videos of the online course (udemy.com: "Explicando la migraña", "Explaining Migraine").

- I fill my head with new information from Arturo Goicoechea.

DISTRACTIONS

- I do hypopressive abs (requires concentration on breathing).

- I go for a walk.

- I do things I like.

- I cook.

- I do housework. When I'm distracted, when I see the pain starting to come and go, I think the brain is already doubting and that's a good sign. And that's when I see it's going to end.

DISAGREEING

- I focus on what I'm doing.

- I don't cancel plans, I make more.

- I meditate.

- "The more it hurts me, the more I move, I look at the sun, I turn up the music... even though I get tears of pain (...), because none of that is a reason for my head to hurt."

- I act like nothing's happening.

TALKING TO THE BRAIN "UNTIL LOGIC WINS"

- "Nothing is attacking me."

- "Go protect the sick!"

- "Pain does not equal damage."

- "There's no physical reason to produce alertness and pain."

- "It's okay."

- "Just because an alarm goes off doesn't mean there's a fire going on."

- "It's not a migraine, it's an evaluative error."

- "There's no danger."

- "I'm totally healthy."

- "I don't need you to protect me anymore."

- "False alarm, no damage done!"
- "Easy, brain."
- I laugh: "Come on, it's all right!"
- "Don't make erroneous evaluations."
- "The pain will pass, because there's no point in it appearing."

WAYS TO "TALK TO THE BRAIN"

- Thinking it.
- Saying it out loud.
- Saying it out loud in front of a mirror.
- Saying it out loud while touching my head.
- Writing.
- Making someone else talk to my brain.

CALMING DOWN

- I try not to let the anxiety get the better of me. I stay calm.
- I lose my fear of pain.
- I downplay pain.
- I avoid negative or fearful intrusive thoughts.

- I don't worry too much.

- I ask someone else to tell me that everything is fine, that there is no harm.

- I convince myself there's no harm.

- I laugh at what's going on.

- I think it's a passing thing.

TAKING THE PILL

- I realize that, whether I take the pill or not, the pain eventually subsides.

- Knowing that nothing serious is going to happen if I don't take the pill. If it doesn't go away, we'll see what we do.

IMAGINATION/VISUALIZATIONS

- I visualize a cord in my brain that sparks and kills the focus of pain.

- I've got photos on my cell phone of cervicals and healthy heads, neurons, synapses.

- I imagine situations in which I normally have a migraine, but without it, being happy and fearless.

- I imagine the head with a helmet.

- I imagine my brain being healthy.

- I imagine the "apoptosis" of nature, the falling of the leaves.

- I imagine in the brain a blank screen where nothing happens.

HABITUATION TO TRIGGERS

- I eat everything and I think it doesn't have to hurt me.

- I stop wearing sunglasses.

- I turn up the music in the car and sing my lungs out.

- I take a deep breath, even if there's a strong odor.

- I go out into the street without fear.

In short, they are ways to avoid fear, laugh at the brain absurdity, give the finger to sensitizing information.

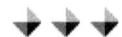

References

1. Anne Carson. Plainwater: Essays and Poetry.; 2000.

2. Fernandes D, Carvalho AL. Mechanisms of homeostatic plasticity in the excitatory synapse. J Neurochem. 2016. doi:10.1111/jnc.13687

3. Ramachandran VS, Bakeslee S, Sacks O. Phantoms in the Brain: Probing the Mysteries of the Human Mind.; 1999.

4. Mittinty MM, Vanlint S, Stocks N, Mittinty MN, Moseley GL. Exploring effect of pain education on chronic pain patients' expectation of recovery and pain intensity. Scand J Pain. 2018. doi:10.1515/sjpain-2018-0023

5. Richter M, Eck J, Straube T, Miltner WHR, Weiss T. Do words hurt? Brain activation during the processing of pain-related words. Pain. 2010. doi:10.1016/j.pain.2009.08.009

6. Burnett D. El Cerebro Idiota: Un Neurocientífico Nos Explica Las Imperfecciones de Nuestra Materia Gris.; 2016.

7. Raichle ME, Gusnard DA. Appraising the brain's energy budget. Proc Natl Acad Sci U S A. 2002. doi:10.1073/pnas.172399499

8. Raichle ME. The restless brain: How intrinsic activity organizes brain function. Philos Trans R Soc B Biol Sci. 2015. doi:10.1098/rstb.2014.0172

9. Colloca L. Nocebo effects can make you feel pain. Science (80 —). 2017. doi:10.1126/science.aap8488

10. Dodick DW. A Phase-by-Phase Review of Migraine Pathophysiology. Headache. 2018. doi:10.1111/head.13300

11. Charles A. Migraine: a brain state. Curr Opin Neurol. 2013. doi:10.1097/WCO.0b013e32836085f4

12. Gelfand AA. Migraine and childhood periodic syndromes in children and adolescents. Curr Opin Neurol. 2013. doi:10.1097/WCO.0b013e32836085c7

13. Grace PM, Hutchinson MR, Maier SF, Watkins LR. Pathological pain and the neuroimmune interface. Nat Rev Immunol. 2014. doi:10.1038/nri3621

14. Pinho-Ribeiro FA, Verri WA, Chiu IM. Nociceptor Sensory Neuron–Immune Interactions in Pain and Inflammation. Trends Immunol. 2017. doi:10.1016/j.it.2016.10.001

15. Mehle ME. Migraine and allergy: A review and clinical update. Curr Allergy Asthma Rep. 2012. doi:10.1007/s11882-012-0251-x

16. Maniyar FH, Sprenger T, Schankin C, Goadsby PJ. The origin of nausea in migraine–A PET study. J Headache Pain. 2014. doi:10.1186/1129-2377-15-84

17. Burgos-Vega C, Moy J, Dussor G. Meningeal afferent signaling and the pathophysiology of migraine. In: Progress in Molecular Biology and Translational Science. ; 2015. doi:10.1016/bs.pmbts.2015.01.001

18. Goadsby PJ, Holland PR, Martins-Oliveira M, Hoffmann J, Schankin C, Akerman S. Pathophysiology of Migraine: A Disorder of Sensory Processing. Physiol Rev. 2017. doi:10.1152/physrev.00034.2015

19. Schoonman GG, Van Der Grond J, Kortmann C, Van Der Geest RJ, Terwindt GM, Ferrari MD. Migraine headache is not associated with cerebral or meningeal vasodilatation — A 3T magnetic resonance angiography study. Brain. 2008. doi:10.1093/brain/awn094

20. Schulte LH, May A. Of generators, networks and migraine attacks. Curr Opin Neurol. 2017. doi:10.1097/WCO.0000000000000441

21. PENFIELD W, BOLDREY E. SOMATIC MOTOR AND

SENSORY REPRESENTATION IN THE CEREBRAL COR-TEX OF MAN AS STUDIED BY ELECTRICAL STIMULA-TION. Brain. 1937. doi:10.1093/brain/60.4.389

22.   Mirza AF, Mo J, Holt JL, et al. Is There a Relationship between Throbbing Pain and Arterial Pulsations? J Neurosci. 2012. doi:10.1523/jneurosci.0193-12.2012

23.   Mo J, Maizels M, Ding M, Ahn AH. Does throbbing pain have a brain signature? Pain. 2013. doi:10.1016/j.pain.2013.02.013

24.   Childs BG, Baker DJ, Kirkland JL, Campisi J, van Deursen JM. Senescence and apoptosis: dueling or complementary cell fates? EMBO Rep. 2014. doi:10.15252/embr.201439245

25.   Roh JS, Sohn DH. Damage-Associated Molecular Patterns in Inflammatory Diseases. Immune Netw. 2018. doi:10.4110/in.2018.18.e27

26.   Woolf CJ, Ma Q. Nociceptors-Noxious Stimulus Detectors. Neuron. 2007. doi:10.1016/j.neuron.2007.07.016

27.   C L, K Y, A B, D K. Migraine-like headache in bacterial meningitis. Cephalalgia. 2000. doi:10.1111/j.1468-2982.2000.00110.x

28.   Moseley GL, Butler DS. Fifteen Years of Explaining Pain: The Past, Present, and Future. J Pain. 2015. doi:10.1016/j.jpain.2015.05.005

29.   Garcia-Larrea L. The posterior insular-opercular region and the search of a primary cortex for pain. Neurophysiol Clin. 2012. doi:10.1016/j.neucli.2012.06.001

30.   Garcia-Larrea L, Peyron R. Pain matrices and neuropathic pain matrices: A review. In: Pain. ; 2013. doi:10.1016/j.pain.2013.09.001

31.   Godinho F, Faillenot I, Perchet C, Frot M, Magnin M, Garcia-Larrea L. How the pain of others enhances our pain: Searching the cerebral correlates of 'compassional hyperalgesia.' Eur J Pain. 2011. doi:10.1002/j.1532-2149.2011.00039.x

32.   Hougaard A, Amin F, Hauge AW, Ashina M, Olesen J. Provocation of migraine with aura using natural trigger factors.

Neurology. 2013. doi:10.1212/WNL.0b013e31827f0f10

33. Goadsby PJ, Silberstein SD. Migraine triggers: Harnessing the messages of clinical practice. Neurology. 2013. doi:10.1212/WNL.0b013e31827f100c

34. Martin PR. Managing headache triggers: Think "coping" not "avoidance." Cephalalgia. 2010. doi:10.1111/j.1468-2982.2009.01989.x

35. Martin PR, Reece J, Callan M, et al. Behavioral management of the triggers of recurrent headache: A randomized controlled trial. Behav Res Ther. 2014. doi:10.1016/j.brat.2014.07.002

36. Malfliet A, Kregel J, Coppieters I, et al. Effect of pain neuroscience education combined with cognition-targeted motor control training on chronic spinal pain a randomized clinical trial. JAMA Neurol. 2018. doi:10.1001/jamaneurol.2018.0492

37. Abraham A. The imaginative mind. Hum Brain Mapp. 2016. doi:10.1002/hbm.23300

38. Marchetti G. Consciousness: a unique way of processing information. Cogn Process. 2018. doi:10.1007/s10339-018-0855-8

39. Noel M, Beals-Erickson SE, Law EF, Alberts NM, Palermo TM. Characterizing the pain narratives of parents of youth with chronic pain. Clin J Pain. 2016. doi:10.1097/AJP.0000000000000346

40. Evans RW, Lipton RB, Silberstein SD. The prevalence of migraine in neurologists. Neurology. 2003. doi:10.1212/01.WNL.0000090628.46508.D4

41. Alstadhaug KB, Hernandez A, Næss H, Stovner LJ. Migraine among Norwegian neurologists. Headache. 2012. doi:10.1111/j.1526-4610.2012.02216.x

42. Waters WE. Migraine in general practitioners. Br J Prev Soc Med. 1975. doi:10.1136/jech.29.1.48

43. Porreca F, Navratilova E. Reward, motivation, and emotion of pain and its relief. Pain. 2017. doi:10.1097/j.pain.0000000000000798

44.   Auvray M, Myin E, Spence C. The sensory-discriminative
      and affective-motivational aspects of pain. Neurosci Biobe-
      hav Rev. 2010. doi:10.1016/j.neubiorev.2008.07.008
{Bibliography}

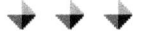

www.ingramcontent.com/pod-product-compliance
Lightning Source LLC
Chambersburg PA
CBHW060854170526
45158CB00001B/351